Non-invasive Respiratory Support

Edited by

Anita K. Simonds

Consultant in Respiratory Medicine
Royal Brompton Hospital
London

CHAPMAN & HALL MEDICAL
London · Glasgow · Weinheim · New York · Tokyo · Melbourne · Madras

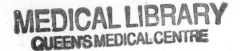
Chapman & Hall, 2–6 Boundary Row, London SE1 8HN, UK

Chapman & Hall, 2–6 Boundary Row, London SE1 8HN, UK

Blackie Academic & Professional, Wester Cleddens Road, Bishopbriggs, Glasgow G64 2NZ, UK

Chapman & Hall GmbH, Pappelallee 3, 69469 Weinheim, Germany

Chapman & Hall USA, 115 Fifth Avenue, New York, NY 10003, USA

Chapman & Hall Japan, ITP-Japan, Kyowa Building, 3F, 2-2-1 Hirakawacho, Chiyoda-ku, Tokyo 102, Japan

Chapman & Hall Australia, 102 Dodds Street, South Melbourne, Victoria 3205, Australia

Chapman & Hall India, R. Seshadri, 32 Second Main Road, CIT East, Madras 600 035, India

First edition 1996

© 1996   Chapman & Hall

Typeset in 10/12 Palatino by Best-set Typesetter Ltd., Hong Kong

Printed in Great Britain by the Alden Press, Oxford

ISBN   0 412 56840 3

A catalogue record for this book is available from the British Library

Library of Congress Catalog Card Number: 95-70878

∞ Printed on permanent acid-free text paper, manufactured in accordance with ANSI/NISO Z39.48-1992 and ANSI/NISO Z39.48-1984 (Permanence of Paper).

Non-invasive Respiratory Support

Contents

Contents

vi

Contributors

Julia Bott, MCSP
Head of Research and Development,
Physiotherapy Department,
Royal Brompton Hospital,
Sydney Street,
London SW3 6NP
UK

Mark W. Elliott, MD, MRCP
Consultant Physician,
St James's University Hospital,
Beckett Street,
Leeds LS9 7TF
UK

John C. Goldstone, MD, FRCA
Senior Lecturer in Anaesthesia,
Consultant in Intensive Care Medicine,
Room 103,
The Middlesex Hospital,
Mortimer Street,
London W1A 8AA
UK

Patrick Leger, MD
Service de Reanimation Medicale et
Assistance Respiratoire,
Hopital de la Croix Rousse,
93 grande rue de la Croix Rousse,
69317 Lyon,
France

Fidelma Moran BSc, MCSP
Senior Physiotherapist,
Mater Misericordiae Hospital,
Dublin,
Ireland

Anita K. Simonds, MD, FRCP
Consultant in Respiratory Medicine,
Royal Brompton Hospital,
Sydney Street,
London SW3 6NP
UK

Preface

In the past decade the area of non-invasive respiratory support has received a tremendous boost from the discovery of novel techniques and new indications for treatment. Underlying these developments is a major increase in knowledge of the effects of sleep on respiration. While negative pressure ventilation will remain useful for some patients, there has been an explosion in the use of nasal intermittent positive pressure ventilation (NIPPV) both for domiciliary purposes and for hospital patients with acute respiratory failure. The obstructive sleep apnoea syndrome is now recognized as an important public health issue, and the treatment of choice for many individuals with this condition is nasal continuous positive airway pressure (CPAP) therapy.

In this book practical aspects of nasal intermittent positive pressure ventilation, negative pressure ventilation, CPAP, and other non-invasive respiratory support methods in adults and children are described, and the indications for treatment outlined. Considerably more space is devoted to NIPPV in the management of acute and chronic ventilatory failure as this mode of non-invasive ventilatory support is likely to be most widely available. The pathophysiology of the underlying conditions and alternatives to non-invasive respiratory support are discussed in some detail as the successful application of any therapy depends not only to knowing *how* to apply it, but also *when* to apply it, and *why* it works.

The essential components of a home care scheme, and patterns of respiratory home care in the United Kingdom, USA and Europe, are considered in the final chapters.

A.K.S.

Abbreviations

ABG	arterial blood gas (tensions)
A/C	assist-control mode ventilation
AHI	apnoea/hypopnoea index
BE	base excess
Ccw	chest wall compliance
Cl	lung compliance
CMD	congenital muscular dystrophy
COPD	chronic obstructive pulmonary disease
CPAP	continuous positive airway pressure
CRI	chronic respiratory insufficiency
DL_{CO}	gas transfer factor
DMD	Duchenne muscular dystrophy
EEG	electroencephalogram
EEPoes	end expiratory oesophageal pressure
EHFO	external high frequency oscillation
EMG	electromyogram
EOG	electro-oculogram
EPAP	expiratory positive airway pressure
$EtCO_2$	end-tidal CO_2
FET	forced expiration technique
FLS	forward lean sitting
FVC	forced vital capacity
HMV	home mechanical ventilation
HRC	home respiratory care
IPAP	inspiratory positive airway pressure
IPPB	intermittent positive pressure breathing
IPPV	intermittent positive pressure ventilation
IPS	inspiratory pressure support
K_{CO}	gas transfer coefficient
LAUP	laser-assisted uvulopalatoplasty
LGMD	limb girdle muscular dystrophy
MV	minute volume
NIPPV	nasal intermittent positive pressure ventilation
MIPPV	mouth(piece) intermittent positive pressure ventilation
MND	motor neurone disease
nPV	negative pressure ventilation
OSA	obstructive sleep apnoea
PE_{max}	maximum expiratory muscle pressure
PEP	positive expiratory pressure
PEEP	positive end expiratory pressure
$PEEP_i$	intrinsic positive end expirating pressure
PI_{max}	maximum inspiratory muscle strength
Poes	oesophageal pressure
SaO_2	arterial oxygen saturation
SIMV	synchronized intermittent mandatory ventilation
SMA	spinal muscular atrophy
SONI	strapless oral nasal interface
S/T	spontaneous/timed ventilation
$TcCO_2$	transcutaneous partial pressure of CO_2
TE	expiratory time
TENS	transcutaneous electrical nerve stimulation
TI	inspiratory time

T-IPPV	tracheostomy intermittent positive pressure ventilation	UVPP	uvulopalatopharyngoplasty
		V_T	tidal volume

1

Modes of non-invasive ventilatory support

ANITA K. SIMONDS

INTRODUCTION

Spontaneous ventilation can be assisted or replaced by delivering intermittent positive pressure to the airway or applying intermittent negative pressure to the chest wall. Ventilatory methods are described as invasive if the airway is intubated, or internal placement of electrodes is required, as in diaphragm pacing. Non-invasive methods avoid airway intubation and are therefore not suitable in individuals with impaired airway reflexes, excessive bronchial secretions or complete ventilatory dependence. The various methods may be listed as follows.

1. Non-invasive

   (a) Positive pressure
       (i) Nasal mask
       (ii) Facemask
       (iii) Nasal plugs
       (iv) Mouthpiece
   (b) Negative pressure
       (i) Iron lung
       (ii) Cuirass
       (iii) Pneumojacket

2. Invasive

   (a) Tracheostomy

   (b) Diaphragm pacing

3. Ventilatory adjuncts

   (a) Pneumobelt
   (b) Rocking bed

It is the non-invasive ventilatory techniques which form the subject of this book.

The concept of applying ventilatory support non-invasively has always been attractive, and the development of these techniques preceded that of airway intubation and intermittent positive pressure ventilation. The initial stimulus for experimentation with both negative pressure ventilation and mask ventilation was to resuscitate infants and individuals saved from drowning. Subsequently, the severe worldwide poliomyelitis outbreaks in the first half of the twentieth century proved a major motivating factor. Many patients who would have previously died from the acute effects of poliomyelitis on the respiratory muscles survived, but required continued ventilatory support in the home. Non invasive techniques evolved to meet this need and now the wheel has turned full circle with non-invasive techniques being used increasingly in acute care situations.

Non-Invasive Respiratory Support. Edited by Anita Simonds. Published by Chapman & Hall, London. ISBN 0412 56840 3.

HISTORICAL DEVELOPMENT OF NEGATIVE PRESSURE VENTILATION

Woollam [1] cites the Scotsman John Dalziel as the first to construct a tank ventilator (or 'iron lung') in 1832. Similar ideas flourished elsewhere in Europe and the USA, with Hauke describing a cabinet-type ventilator in Austria in 1874. Dr Alfred Jones of Kentucky patented the first American tank ventilator in 1864. These early workers advocated the use of negative pressure respiration in a myriad of conditions including asphyxia, atelectasis, croup, diphtheria, bronchitis, seminal weakness and paralysis! It is interesting to note that Hauke and his coworker, Waldenburg, were also among the first to use continuous positive airway pressure via a facemask to treat pneumonia and atelectasis. Earlier, in 1854 Woillez in France had outlined the principles of artificial ventilation. In 1876 he produced the Spiropore, a tank ventilator with a remarkable resemblance to twentieth-century models. Bellows were used to evacuate air from a metal cylinder which encased the patient's body. Sporadic developments continued over the next 50 years, but it was not until the 1930s that negative pressure ventilation (nPV) was put to extensive use.

Drinker and colleagues reported an improved iron lung system in 1928. This had an effective airtight seal and portholes to observe the patient and incorporated a sphygmomanometer and stethoscope. According to Woollam [2], this equipment was first demonstrated in the UK in 1931, prompting brisk correspondence in *The Lancet* of that year. Subsequent versions include the Both wooden cabinet respirator, and a rotating model designed by Kelleher to facilitate physiotherapy and postural drainage.

Parallel to the evolution of the iron lung, more portable negative pressure devices were being developed. Hauke used a metal cuirass to enclose the anterior part of the chest in adults and children in the 1870s. The brilliant innovator Alexander Graham Bell devised a negative pressure jacket with the aim of suporting ventilation in premature infants in 1881. This was used with apparent success to resuscitate drowned cats, but its potential was not recognized by the scientific community. Early versions of the cuirass were evacuated with a foot-powered bellows pump. Eisenmenger in Hungary devised a motorized fan extraction system in 1927. Further practical modifications, the Sahlin–Stille cuirass and Burstall jacket, appeared in the 1930s. These models were made of metal and therefore cumbersome and inflexible. This deficiency was overcome with the introduction of plastic or polyurethane shells and jacket devices comprising nylon garment secured over a lightweight frame (e.g. Tunnicliffe jacket, Emerson wrap and pneumosuit).

There was a major poliomyelitis outbreak in the UK in 1938. The pressing need for widely available ventilatory support was recognized by the Medical Research Council. As a result, negative pressure tank ventilators were distributed throughout the UK and the Empire, the equipment being financed by Lord Nuffield. In their observations on the use of respirators in poliomyelitis, Plum and Wolff [3] found the tank ventilator to be the safest device for managing ventilatory insufficiency, but cautioned against overventilation. They found that the cuirass used in the acute phase of the illness was too inefficient.

The American Council on Physical Medicine in 1947 examined the efficiency of the nPV equipment then available and issued an outline of requirements for future cuirass systems. Many of the problems identified by this report and other studies that followed [4,5] are familiar to recent workers in the field and were re-investigated in the 1980s.

Although the use of nPV undoubtedly saved many lives, mortality from acute poliomyelitis remained high, even after the introduction of tracheostomy for bulbar paralysis

in 1943 and the modification of tank ventilators to incorporate tracheostomized cases.
Larssen and Ibsen introduced manual intermittent positive pressure ventilation during
an overwhelming polio epidemic in Copen-
hagen in 1952. This development halved
previous mortality rates and saw the rapid
replacement of negative pressure by positive
pressure techniques.

With the wane in use of nPV (apart from its
use in some convalescent polio patients), indications for its application changed to more
chronic respiratory disorders. Bourteline-
Young and Whittenberger [6] in 1951 describe
the use of the tank ventilator in two patients
with end-stage emphysema. One patient
experienced a rapid correction of arterial
blood gas tensions after a short period of
negative pressure ventilation and improvement was maintained a year later. Success
was attributed to the resetting of respiratory
drive following correction of hypercapnia.
No benefit was seen in the second patient
who, notably, had a history of bronchiectasis
and recurrent wheeze. In 1963 the short-term
effects of nPV using a body suit (Emerson
wrap) was studied in a further group of patients with emphysema and CO_2 retention
[7]. Synchronization of the negative pressure
pump was achieved by sensing a drop in
intranasal or tracheostomy pressure. In stable
patients the use of nPV resulted in a fall in
$PaCO_2$ and correction of acidosis. Less marked
changes were seen in patients with an acute
exacerbation of chronic obstructive pulmonary disease. Trials of nPV in COPD in the
1960s and 1970s produced mixed results [8,9].

RECENT APPLICATIONS OF nPV

With the recognition of the influence of respiratory muscle weakness and physiological
changes during sleep on the pathogenesis of
ventilatory failure, negative pressure techniques were re-explored in the early 1980s
[10,11]. Pneumosuits or negative pressure

jackets were favoured for home use by many
centres, although tailor-made cuirasses and
more portable iron lungs continued to be
employed in patients with chest wall and
neuromuscular disease. The outcome of these
techniques in restrictive and obstructive ventilatory disorders is described in detail in
Chapters 8 and 9.

PNEUMOBELT

The original version of the pneumobelt, the
Bragg–Paul Pulsator, was devised by the
physicist William Bragg in 1938. He is said to
have created the system from several rubber
football bladders which were placed around
the abdomen and lower thorax and inflated
to aid expiration [2].

THE ROCKING BED

The novel employement of a rocking bed to
facilitate diaphragm excursion was described
by Eve [12] in an article titled 'Actuation of
the inert diaphragm by gravity method' in
1932. Here gravity-assisted movement of the
abdominal contents is used to displace the
diaphragm. In poliomyelitis outbreaks a fast
rocking bed was used at rates of up to 24
oscillations a minute, rotating through an arc
of 20 degrees from the horizontal. It was
found to be of most value in the recovery
phase of the disease. However, in some patients the rocking bed was able to delay the
need for more intensive ventilation and aid
weaning [3].

NON-INVASIVE POSITIVE PRESSURE
TECHNIQUES

MASK CPAP/VENTILATION

Masks have a long track record of use to aid
resuscitation or deliver gaseous anaesthetics.
Contionous positive airway pressure (CPAP)
used via a facemask has a role in treating

3

hypoxaemia due to acute conditions such as pulmonary oedema, pneumonia and atelectasis, and may also reduce the work of breathing [13] and sleep disordered breathing [14] in patients with respiratory insufficiency due to COPD.

Sullivan and colleagues [15] in 1981 recognized the value of nasal CPAP in the treatment of obstructive sleep apnoea (OSA) (Chapter 13). Mask CPAP therapy for OSA was the springboard to development of nasal intermittent positive pressure ventilation (NIPPV) for patients with chronic ventilatory failure. The techniques of CPAP and NIPPV are, of course, different despite the fact that similar facemasks or nasal masks can be employed. During CPAP patients continue to breathe spontaneously at their own rate and depth, whereas during NIPPV minute ventilation is augmented with gas flow being determined predominantly by the ventilator. Bi-level pressure support can also be delivered by mask. Airway pressure profiles for CPAP, NIPPV and bi-level pressure support ventilation are displayed in Fig. 1.1.

Since its introduction in the 1980s there has been a very rapid uptake of NIPPV in Europe and the USA for patients requiring home ventilatory support. Figure 1.2 shows the

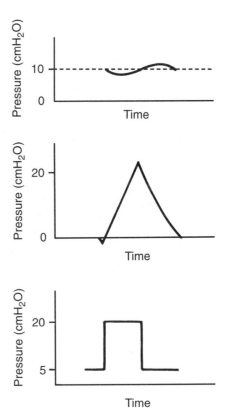

Fig. 1.1 Pressure profiles of continuous positive airway pressure (CPAP) (*top*), triggered nasal entilation (*middle*) and bi-level positive pressure support ventilation (*bottom*).

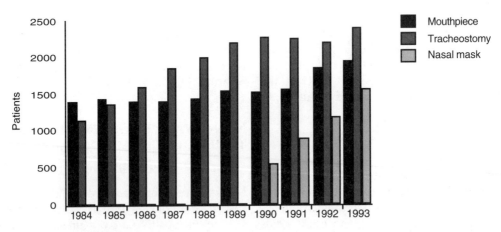

Fig. 1.2 Trends in assisted ventilation in France, 1984–1993 (Data from ANTADIR with permission).

growth in number of patients in France using NIPPV in comparison to other methods of ventilatory support, including tracheostomy-IPPV. NIPPV was first applied to patients with neuromuscular disorders and chest wall disease and use has now extended to some subgroups with chronic obstructive lung disease. The results of NIPPV in these patients are given in Chapters 8 and 9.

MOUTH VENTILATION

Intermittent positive pressure breathing (IPPB) was used widely as a therapy for COPD several decades ago, but declined in use when benefit over and above standard nebulized use could not be confirmed [16]. Mouthpiece intermittent positive pressure ventilation (MIPPV) is used for some patients with COPD, particularly in France [17], but has a more closely defined role in neuromuscular patients with minimal ventilatory capacity [4,18,19].

REFERENCES

1. Woollam, C.H.M. (1976) The development of apparatus for intermittent negative pressure respiration (1) 1832–1918. *Anaesthesia*, **31**, 537–47.
2. Woollam, C.H.M. (1976) The development of apparatus for intermittent negative pressure respiration (2) 1919–1976. *Anaesthesia*, **31**, 666–85.
3. Plum, F. and Wolff, H.G. (1951) Observations on acute poliomyelitis with respiratory insufficiency. *J. Am. Med. Assoc.*, **146**, 442–6.
4. Sortor, S. (1992) Pulmonary issues in quadriplegia. *Eur. Respir. Rev.*, **2**(10), 330–4.
5. Bryce-Smith, R. and Davis, H.S. (1954) Tidal exchange in respirators. *Curr. Res. Anaesth. Analg.*, **33**, 73–85.
6. Bourteline-Young, H.G. and Whittenberger, J.L. (1951) The use of artificial respiration in pulmonary emphysema accompanied by high carbon dioxide levels. *J. Clin. Invest.*, **30**, 838–46.
7. Marks, A., Bocles, J. and Morganti, L. (1963) A new ventilatory assistor for patients with respiratory acidosis. *N. Engl. J. Med.*, **268**, 61–8.
8. McClement, J., Christianson, L.C. and Hubaytor, R.T. (1965) The body type respirator in the treatment of chronic obstructive pulmonary disease. *Ann. NY Acad. Sci.*, **121**, 748.
9. Fountain, F.F., Reynolds, L.B. and Tickle, S.M. (1973) Use of extrathoracic assisted breathing in the management of chronic obstructive lung disease. *Am. J. Phys. Med.*, **52**, 277–88.
10. Braun, N.M.T. (1985) Effect of daily intermittent rest on respiratory muscles on patients with CAO. *Chest*, **85**, 595–605.
11. Garay, S.M., Turino, G.M. and Goldring, R.M. (1981) Sustained reversal of chronic hypercapnia in patients with alveolar hypoventilation syndromes. *Am. J. Med.*, **70**, 269–74.
12. Eve, F.G. (1932) Actuation of inert diaphragm by gravity method. *Lancet*, **2**, 995–7.
13. Petrof, B.J., Legare, M., Goldberg, P. *et al.* (1990) Continuous positive airway pressure reduces work of breathing and dyspnea during weaning from mechanical ventilation in severe chronic obstructive pulmonary disease. *Am. Rev. Respir. Dis.*, **141**, 281–9.
14. Petrof, B.J., Kimoff, R.J., Levy, R.D. *et al.* (1991) Nasal continuous positive airway pressure facilitates respiratory muscle function during sleep in severe chronic obstructive pulmonary disease. *Am. Rev. Respir. Dis.*, **143**, 928–35.
15. Sullivan, C.E., Issa, F.G., Berthon-Jones, M. and Eves, L. (1981) Reversal of obstructive sleep apnea by continuous positive pressure applied through the nares. *Lancet*, **1**, 862–5.
16. The Intermittent Positive Pressure Breathing Trial Group (1983) Intermittent positive pressure breathing therapy of chronic obstructive pulmonary disease. *Ann. Intern. Med.*, **99**, 612–20.
17. Muir, J.-F. (1992) Intermittent positive pressure ventilation (IPPV) in patients with chronic obstructive pulmonary disease (COPD). *Eur. Respir. Rev.*, **2**(10), 335–45.

18. Bach, J.R., Alba, A.S., Bohatiuk, G. *et al.* (1987) Mouth intermittent positive pressure ventilation in the management of postpolio respiratory insufficiency. *Chest*, **91**, 859–64.

19. Bach, J.R., Alba, A.S. and Saporito, L.R. (1993) Intermittent positive pressure ventilation via the mouth as an alternative to tracheostomy for 257 ventilator users. *Chest*, **103**, 174–82.

Pathophysiology of ventilatory failure

ANITA K. SIMONDS

INTRODUCTION

The adequacy of ventilation is dependent on an intact chain of command which extends from the brain via the effector muscles to the alveolus. From a conceptual point of view, it is helpful to appreciate that ventilatory failure will occur when the load placed on the respiratory system exceeds the capacity to accommodate this, or ventilatory drive is inadequate [1]. The balance between load, capacity and drive is crucial. It follows that conditions which increase ventilatory load, reduce ventilatory capacity or impair drive will place the individual at risk of respiratory insufficiency. The interplay of these factors in chronic obstructive lung disease is shown in Fig. 2.1. In health, a considerable degree of respiratory reserve exists so that changes in load, for example, increased lower airways resistance due to asthma, are well tolerated. However, where the balance between load and capacity is precarious, minor alterations may precipitate respiratory decompensation. Of particular importance are the physiological changes which take place during sleep. Here, fluctuations in central drive, respiratory muscle function, airway tone and responses to load can lead to nocturnal hypoventilation and ultimately diurnal respiratory failure. This sequence of events explains the rationale of nocturnal monitoring of respiration in susceptible individuals, and the use of ventilatory support during sleep in those with hypercapnic respiratory failure.

The causes of increased ventilatory load, reduced capacity and ventilatory drive defects are listed in Fig. 2.2, and described below with particular reference to pathophysiological features in COPD, chest wall disease and neuromuscular disorders.

CONTROL OF BREATHING

Breathing is controlled by a system that is required to regulate hydrogen ion concentration, PaO_2 and $PaCO_2$, while at the same time accommodating functions such as swallowing and speech. Inspiratory activity generated in the brain stem is modified by afferent input from central and peripheral chemoreceptors, plus feedback from vagal and upper airway receptors which respond to stretch and pressure. Abnormal control of breathing may result from lesions to the pons or medulla, primary or acquired reductions in chemosensitivity to $PaCO_2$ and PaO_2, or defective information from mechanoreceptors. In addition, there are diurnal changes in control mechanisms.

During sleep, overall ventilation decreases.

Non-Invasive Respiratory Support. Edited by Anita Simonds. Published by Chapman & Hall, London. ISBN 0412 56840 3.

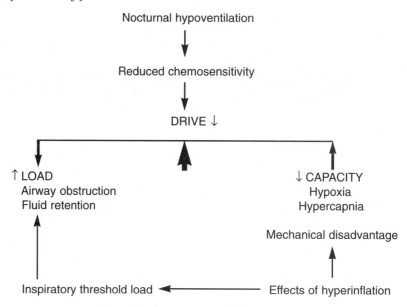

Fig. 2.1 Interactions between ventilatory load, capacity and drive in COPD (Courtesy M, Elliott).

This is due to a reduction in cortical stimulation of the respiratory centres (wakefulness drive) [2], and a diminution in chemosensitivity to $PaCO_2$ and PaO_2. Changes in $PaCO_2$ and arterial oxygen saturation are most marked during phasic periods of REM sleep. Measurement of drive during REM sleep is fraught with problems as steady state conditions do not apply. However, examination of the minute ventilation response to hypercapnia has confirmed that both the slope and position of the CO_2 response curve alter during sleep [3]. As these results may be compounded by variable contributions from the respiratory muscles, Hubmayr and colleagues [4] have examined the CO_2 recruitment threshold in patients in whom the respiratory muscles were unloaded (and therefore inactive) using non-invasive ventilation. In normal subjects the level of $PaCO_2$ at which spontaneous ventilation was initiated was 38 mmHg when awake and around 41–42 mmHg in NREM and REM sleep. Hypoxic drive falls during sleep, reaching a nadir in REM periods [5].

CONGENITAL DRIVE DISORDERS

Congenital absence of ventilatory drive (Ondine's curse) is rare. Here failure of automatic control of breathing results in profound hypoventilation as voluntary control of breathing ceases at the onset of sleep. Blood gases are usually abnormal during the day. Cases are diagnosed in the neonatal period and may be complicated by central disorders such as aberrant temperature control and autonomic instability. Ventilatory support is invariably required – there is no role for respiratory stimulants. Some children are successfully treated by diaphragm pacing but a tracheostomy is usually required in this situation to avoid inducing upper airway obstruction (see Chapter 12).

ACQUIRED DISORDERS OF VENTILATORY DRIVE

Lesions to the brain stem (e.g. cerebrovascular accident, encephalitis, anoxic brain damage) can produce an acquired form of Ondine's

VENTILATORY CAPACITY

Decreased drive

Reduced respiratory muscle strength
 Phrenic nerve weakness
 Myopathy
 Muscular dystrophy
 Myasthenia
 Malnutrition
 Endoncrinopathy
 Hypoxaemia, hypercapnia, acidosis
 Hypophosphataemia
 Hyperinflation
 Disuse atrophy

VENTILATORY LOAD

 High metabolic rate
 Increased deadspace ventilation
 Airways resistance
 Hyperinflation
 Chest wall deformity
 Parenchymal lung disease
 Left ventricular failure

Fig. 2.2 Factors affecting ventilatory capacity and load.

curse. The commonest cause of reduction in hypercapnic drive is secondary depression due to chronic hypercapnia which is seen in patients with neuromuscular disease, chest wall disorders and COPD. Sleep deprivation and fragmentation exacerbate the problem by causing further decreases in chemosensitivity [6].

The obesity–hypoventilation syndrome is a term used to describe the development of hypercapnic respiratory failure in severely obese individuals. In many of these patients obtructive sleep apnoea is present; however, around one-quarter demonstrate pure hypoventilation during sleep which is probably the result of ineffective coupling of central drive with the thoracic pump, and acquired drive defects as a result of chronic hypercapnia.

RESPIRATORY MUSCLES

In health the respiratory muscles act in concert to optimize the bellows function of the rib cage and maintain upper airway patency. Recruitment of the respiratory muscles varies during rest and exertion, on changing posture and during sleep. Pathology involving the diaphragm or phrenic nerve has a more profound effect than impairment of other respiratory muscles, as the diaphragm is the most important inspiratory muscle. However, although bilateral diaphragm failure results in orthopnoea and a fall in vital capacity, overt hypercapnic respiratory failure is unusual unless other respiratory muscles are also involved, or there is additional pulmonary or chest wall pathology [1].

The measurement of respiratory muscle strength is described in Chapter 7. In conditions affecting the respiratory muscles respiratory failure is unusual unless respiratory muscle strength falls below 30% of predicted values.

In some clinical situations the respiratory muscles are not weak, but functionally impaired. Static respiratory mouth pressures are reduced in patients with a scoliosis or thoracoplasty. Cooper *et al.* [7] have analysed respiratory mechanics in individuals with adolescent onset idiopathic scoliosis and moderately well-preserved lung volumes (total lung capacity 75% predicted, angle of scoliosis <60°). In this group, maximum inspiratory mouth pressures were reduced whereas values for expiratory muscle strength were normal, suggesting that overall the muscles were not weak but acting at a mechanical disadvantage.

Hyperinflation is a common feature is patients with moderate to severe COPD, or chronic asthma, its presence indicated by a low, flat diaphragm and barrel chest appearance. The efficiency of breathing is reduced by hyperinflation due to a decrease in intrinsic efficiency of the respiratory muscles when functioning at a higher volume and shorter length, and a change in efficiency of respiratory muscle coupling leading to a rise in oxygen consumption and CO_2 production.

Theoretically, fatigue can be produced in any muscle if the load applied to it is sufficient. Fatigue is defined as the loss of capacity to develop force and/or velocity in response to a load, which is reversible by rest [8]. It has been argued that respiratory muscle fatigue is an important factor in the pathogenesis of ventilatory failure, and as a consequence treatment should be logically directed at 'resting' fatigued muscles. However, it now seems likely that adaptive changes occur to prevent the development of fatigue. In support of this, recent work has shown that resting the respiratory muscles in COPD patients with hypercapnic respiratory failure has no beneficial effect on respiratory muscle function [9]. A persuasive hypothesis is that when load exceeds capacity, the onset of peripheral muscle fatigue leads to a reduction in central drive which serves to protect the muscles from further damage [1].

THORACIC PUMP DURING SLEEP

With the transition from wakefulness to sleep there is an overall reduction in skeletal muscle tone. During NREM sleep the relative contribution of the rib cage and abdomen to respiration alter. There appears to be an increase in rib cage excursion [10]. In contrast, during REM sleep much of the tidal volume is generated by the diaphragm due to a marked fall in muscle tone in the intercostal and accessory muscles. This REM-related hypotonia is thought to be a result of either postsynaptic inhibition or a reduction in the activity of presynaptic excitatory neurones.

At the same time, pharyngeal resistance increases and compliance falls due to hypotonia of the upper airway musculature. This rise in upper airway resistance contributes to the decrease in tidal volume and minute ventilation seen during sleep, and leads to overt upper airway obstruction in sleep in predisposed individuals (see Chapter 13).

CHEST WALL CHARACTERISTICS

In chest wall disorders the compliance of the chest wall (Ccw) plays an important role in determining lung volumes and the work of breathing. For patients with idiopathic scoliosis the Cobb angle (a measure of the degree of scoliosis) is inversely related to Ccw. Individuals with a Cobb angle of less than 50° experience a minimal reduction in Ccw whereas in those with a Cobb angle exceeding 50° Ccw is decreased significantly [11]. In subjects with severe respiratory muscle weakness secondary to poliomyelitis (vital capacity between 240 and 1400 ml) chest wall compliance was approximately half that in normal subjects. On a similar note, Kafer [12] found that 50% of ambulant poliomyelitis patients studied had around a 50% reduction in total compliance of the respiratory system.

This alteration in chest wall properties may occur in patients with respiratory muscle weakness without spinal or rib cage deformity. Estenne and colleagues [13] have demonstrated a decrease in Ccw in 75% of patients with chronic respiratory muscle weakness without scoliosis (mean vital capacity 58.7% predicted). A low tidal volume pattern of breathing which fails to fully expand the chest wall (and lungs) is thought to be the cause of this transformation in chest wall mechanical properties.

The integrity of chest wall excursion is affected by paradoxical movement in thoracoplasty (and neuromuscular) patients and this increases the work of breathing. Although positive pressure ventilation can reverse paradoxical movement, the lung beneath any thoracoplasty site is usually damaged and unlikely to take part in normal gas exchange. The effects of a hyperinflated chest on the bellows function of the respiratory muscles have been described earlier (p. 9).

PULMONARY CHARACTERISTICS

CHEST WALL DISORDERS AND NEUROMUSCULAR DISEASE

It is rare to find independent pulmonary pathology in patients with restrictive chest wall disease secondary to scoliosis, although recurrent atelectasis may occur in those with neuromuscular defects. In non-smokers, airway resistance is low and gas trapping uncommon. Gas transfer coefficient (K_{CO}) is often raised in the presence of a low transfer factor (DL_{CO}) in scoliotic patients as extrathoracic compression of the lung squeezes out more air than blood. A low K_{CO} value should raise the suspicion of additional intrapulmonary pathology or pulmonary hypertension. Pulmonary fibrosis is common in patients with previous tuberculosis. Individuals with a thoracoplasty may also have a fixed component of airflow obstruction due, in part, to airway distortion.

Many studies have shown a reduction in lung compliance (Cl) in the majority of patients with scoliosis of a paralytic or idiopathic variety. Changes in Cl are unrelated to age, aetiology of curvature, or history of previous lung infection. Not only are values for Cl low, but the pulmonary pressure–volume curve is shifted to the right. This feature is also seen in patients with respiratory muscle weakness [14], and following experimental strapping of the chest wall in normal subjects [15].

Reduction in Cl can be attributed to several different mechanisms – microatelectasis, a generalized change in alveolar surface forces and/or an alteration in tissue elasticity. Estenne and colleagues [16] have recently investigated the role of microatelectasis in paitents with respiratory muscle weakness using high resolution tomography. The CT scans of 1 mm in thickness showed no parenchymal abnormality in the majority of patiens. Two out of 12 subjects had small areas of atelectasis. Its seems likely therefore that an alteration in alveolar surface forces caused by chronic hypoventilation and underinflation of the alveoli is largely responsible for the fall in Cl. If this were the case, hyperinflation should reverse these changes. Data on this score are conflicting. The alternative possibility of a change in elastic forces has not been demonstrated, but is favoured by some workers [16].

CHRONIC OBSTRUCTIVE PULMONARY DISEASE

Airflow obstruction and uneven ventilation characterize COPD. Blood flow may be patchy because of emphysematous destruction of the pulmonary vascular bed, compression of vessels by alveolar distension and hypoxic vasoconstriction. Hypoxaemia is caused by ventilation–perfusion mismatch and alveolar hypoventilation. Diffusion defects also contribute, the lowest values for gas transfer being seen in emphysematous patients. As indicated above, desaturation is first seen during REM sleep in COPD patients, the most profound hypoxaemic dips occurring in patients with a low SaO_2 during wakefulness (Fig. 2.3). This is because, for a given drop in PO_2, desaturation will be most severe in those who start the night with an SaO_2 on the steep slope of the oxyhaemoglobin dissociation curve. Arterial blood gas derangement during sleep in COPD is primarily a result of hypoventilation due to loss of intercostal and upper airway muscle tone, plus a decrease in ventilatory drive, rather than further changes in ventilation–perfusion relationships, although the latter may contribute.

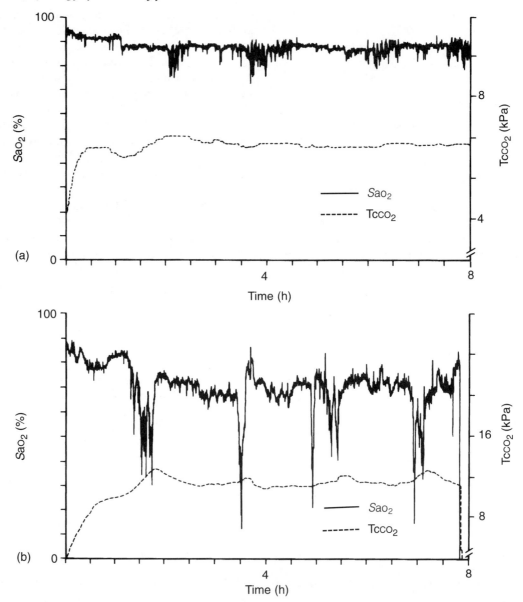

Fig. 2.3 Sleep disordered breathing in COPD: (a) mild, REM-related; (b) severe. $TcCO_2$ = transcutaneous PCO_2.

EVOLUTION OF SLEEP DISORDERED BREATHING

In patients with COPD and neuromusculo-skeletal disorders, mild REM-related hypo-ventilation is often asymptomatic. However, once progression to disturbances in NREM sleep is seen, symptoms are usually manifest, although these are often non-specific feelings

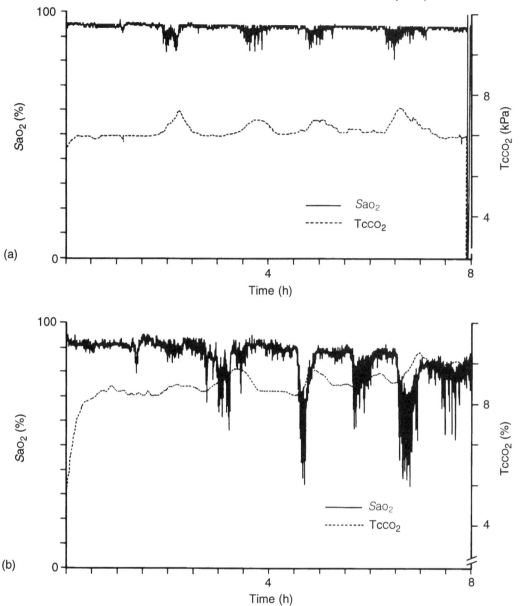

Fig. 2.4 Nocturnal hypoventilation in patient with early onset scoliosis: (a) at ideal body weight; (b) one year later, following weight gain of 8 kg. $Tcco_2$ = transcutaneous Pco_2.

of tiredness, an unrefreshed sensation and headaches on waking. In neuromuscular disorders the rate of progression depends on the extent of involvement of the respiratory muscles. During intercostal and accessory muscle inhibition in REM sleep, virtually the sole muscle of inspiration is the diaphragm so that bilateral early involvement of the dia-

13

phragm will hasten the rate of decline. In all cases a vicious cycle of hypoventilation leading to hypercapnia and secondary depression of hypercapnic ventilatory drive occurs. This may be exacerbated by sleep fragmentation.

It is not clear whether ventilatory responses and respiratory muscle function decline with age. There is evidence that respiratory muscle function may deteriorate, particularly in patients with previous poliomyelitis many years after the initial viral insult. A post-polio syndrome has been described in which muscle function is further compromised by auto-immune mediated damage. Weight gain may tip the balance in an individual with border-line respiratory function. Figure 2.4 shows the progression of sleep disordered breathing in a patient with idiopathic scoliosis who gained 8 kg in weight.

The additional presence of obstructive sleep apnoea will also lead to a greater degree of nocturnal desaturation than might be expected on the basis of lung function and daytime blood gases. Both COPD and obstructive sleep apnoea are common conditions. The combination of OSA and COPD (the overlap syndrome) should always be suspected in COPD patients in whom nocturnal desaturation is disproportionate to spirometry. Bulbar dysfunction can also lead to upper airway obstruction in patients with neuromuscular disorders (e.g. poliomyelitis and Duchenne muscular dystrophy). In some individuals obstructive apnoeas predate nocturnal hypoventilation; in others an upper airway obstructive component and central hypoventilation co-exist (Fig. 2.5).

CONSEQUENCES OF NOCTURNAL AND DIURNAL HYPOVENTILATION

Swings in pulmonary artery pressure have been shown to accompany episodes of hypoxaemia during sleep. Hypercapnia and acidosis probably also contribute. However, it is not clear in any patient with sleep disordered

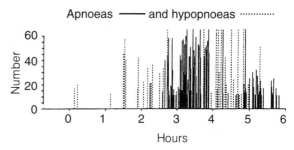

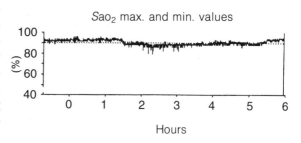

Fig. 2.5 Sleep disordered breathing in patient with previous poliomyelitis. A mixture of obstructive apnoeas (solid lines) and hypopnoeas (dotted lines) is seen.

breathing to what degree nocturnal events and diurnal desaturation on exercise contribute to the development of pulmonary hypertension and cor pulmonale. Responses to nocturnal hypoventilation may differ in restrictive and obstructive disorders. One study of COPD patients has shown that levels of nocturnal hypoxaemia did not improve the prediction of survival over and above wake values of Sao_2 [17]. No such information is available on other groups of patients, such as those with chest wall disease, although many workers in the field have the clear impression that nocturnal hypoventilation gives important prognostic information. However, as these patients also have the most abnormal blood gases by day, no firm conclusions can be drawn. It is important to bear in mind that pulmonary hypertension occurs on exercise in patients with severe restrictive ventilatory defects in the absence of hypoxaemia as there is inadequate vascular bed to accommodate the increased cardiac output [18].

Right ventricular failure was the cause of death in 30% of 102 patients with untreated idiopathic scoliosis followed up for 50 years by Freyschuss and colleagues [19]. Death was premature at the age of 46.6 years for the group. As might be expected, those with the smallest lungs were at the greatest risk of developing cardiorespiratory failure.

REFERENCES

1. Green, M. and Moxham, J. (1993) Respiratory muscles in health and disease, in *Respiratory Medicine: Recent Advances* (ed. P.J. Barnes), Butterworth-Heinemann, Oxford, pp. 252–75.
2. Orem, J. (1994) The wakefulness stimulus for breathing, in *Sleep and Breathing* (eds N.A. Saunders and C.E. Sullivan), Marcel Dekker, New York, pp. 113–55.
3. Douglas, N.J., White, D.P., Weil, J.V. *et al.* (1982) Hypercapnic ventilatory response in sleeping adults. *Am. Rev. Respir. Dis.*, **126**, 758–62.
4. Prechter, G.C., Nelson, S.B. and Hubmayr, R.D. (1990) The ventilatory recruitment threshold for carbon dioxide. *Am. Rev. Respir. Dis.*, **141**, 758–64.
5. Berthon-Jones, M. and Sullivan, C.E. (1982) Ventilatory and arousal responses to hypoxia in sleeping humans. *Am. Rev. Respir. Dis.*, **125**, 632–9.
6. White, D.P., Douglas, N.J., Pickett, C.K. *et al.* (1983) Sleep deprivation and control of ventilation. *Am. Rev. Respir. Dis.*, **128**, 984–6.
7. Cooper, D.M., Rojas, J.V., Mellins, R.B. *et al.* (1984) Respiratory mechanics in adolescents with idiopathic scoliosis. *Am. Rev. Respir. Dis.*, **130**, 16–22.
8. NHLBI Workshop (1990) Respiratory muscle fatigue: report of the respiratory muscle fatigue workshop. *Am. Rev. Respir. Dis.*, **142**, 474–80.
9. Elliott, M.W., Mulvey, D.A., Moxham, J. *et al.* (1991) Domiciliary nocturnal nasal intermittent positive pressure ventilation in COPD: mechanisms underlying changes in arterial blood gas tensions. *Eur. Respir. J.*, **4**, 1044–52.
10. Tabachnik, E., Muller, N.L., Bryan, A.C. and Levison, H. (1981) Changes in ventilation and chest wall mechanics during sleep in normal adolescents. *J. Appl. Physiol.*, **51**, 557–64.
11. Bergofsky, E.H. (1979) Respiratory failure in disorders of the thoracic cage. *Am. Rev. Respir. Dis.*, **119**, 643–69.
12. Kafer, E. (1974) Respiratory function in paralytic scoliosis. *Am. Rev. Respir. Dis.*, **110**, 450–7.
13. Estenne, M., Heilporn, A., Delhez, L. *et al.* (1983) Chest wall stiffness in patients with chronic respiratory muscle weakness. *Am. Rev. Respir. Dis.*, **128**, 1002–7.
14. Gibson, G.J., Pride, N.B., Newsom-Davis, J.N. and Loh, L.C. (1977) Pulmonary mechanics in patients with respiratory muscle weakness. *Am. Rev. Respir. Dis.*, **115**, 389–95.
15. Caro, C.G., Butler, J. and DuBois, A.B. (1960) Some effects of restriction of chest cage expansion on pulmonary function in man: an experimental study. *J. Clin. Invest.*, **39**, 573–83.
16. Kinnear, W., Gevenois, P.A., Estenne, M. and De Troyer, A. (1991) Reduced pulmonary compliance in quadriplegic patients – the role of microatelectasis. *Am. Rev. Respir. Dis.*, **143**, A166.
17. Connaughton, J.J., Catterall, J.R., Elton, R.A. *et al.* (1988) Do sleep studies contribute to the management of patients with severe chronic pulmonary disease? *Am. Rev. Respir. Dis.*, **138**, 341–5.
18. Shneerson, J.M. (1978) Pulmonary artery pressure in thoracic scoliosis during and after exercise while breathing air and pure oxygen. *Thorax*, **33**, 747–54.
19. Freyschuss, V., Nilsonne, U. and Lundgren, K.D. (1968) Idiopathic scoliosis in old age. 1. Respiratory function. *Arch. Med. Scand.*, **184**, 365.

3

Equipment

ANITA K. SIMONDS

INTRODUCTION

A number of factors need to be taken into account when choosing which ventilatory technique is appropriate for the patient. The underlying pathophysiology, degree of ventilator dependency, level of general mobility and preference of the patient should be important considerations. Cost and staff training are likely to remain major factors. The types of ventilatory systems available are described below, divided into the categories of non-invasive positive pressure equipment, negative pressure devices and ventilatory adjuncts.

NON-INVASIVE POSITIVE PRESSURE VENTILATORS

The ideal ventilator for use in mask or face-piece ventilation would have the following characteristics.

- User-friendly.
- Portable/quiet.
- Assist/control.
- Sensitive trigger.
- Reliable and robust.
- Low cost/low maintenance.
- Battery option.
- Low pressure, high pressure and power alarms.

- Humidification facility.
- Can be powered by compressor or piped gas.
- Versatile.
- Capable of ventilating individuals with low and high thoracopulmonary compliance.
- Pressure support option.

Not surprisingly, no such model exists, but some ventilators go a long way to meeting the needs of most patients requiring respiratory support. Most research work has focused on the performance of ventilators employed with nasal masks.

The simplest classification of mask ventilators is into volume-preset and pressure-preset models. The earliest studies of NIPPV employed volume-preset equipment and these are still the most widely used ventilators worldwide. However, pressure-present equipment is gaining ground, particularly in the form of bi-level pressure support systems such as the BiPAP (Respironics) and DP90 (Taema).

VOLUME-PRESET VERSUS PRESSURE-PRESET POSITIVE PRESSURE SYSTEMS

Both volume- and pressure-preset apparatus have advantages and disadvantages in clinical

Non-Invasive Respiratory Support. Edited by Anita Simonds. Published by Chapman & Hall, London. ISBN 0412 56840 3.

practice. Generally, the newer pressure-preset models are smaller and more compact than volume-preset apparatus, but as a consequence they are usually less powerful in terms of flow generation. In theory, volume-preset equipment is able to provide a constant level of alveolar ventilation in the face of changing pulmonary characteristics – for example, in patients with variable bronchospasm or rapidly altering pulmonary compliance. However, they compensate for leaks poorly. In contrast, pressure-preset equipment compensates well for small leaks from around the mask or mouth, but will deliver a reduced minute volume if lung compliance falls or airway resistance increases. For practical purposes, this failure to match the patient's changing ventilatory requirements may only be important in an unstable patient with an acute exacerbation of chronic disease rather than in stable patients receiving home ventilation.

There are few studies comparing volume-preset and pressure-preset ventilators. Elliott *et al.* [1] have examined the effects of nasal ventilation via a pressure support system, with a volume cycled flow generator delivery and continuous positive airway pressure (CPAP). The pressure support system (BiPAP, Respironics Inc.) was used in inspiratory positive airway pressure (IPAP) mode, and inspiratory plus expiratory positive pressure mode (IPAP + EPAP). These forms of ventilatory assistance were randomly applied to 11 stable outpatients with hypercapnic respiratory failure due to chronic obstructive pulmonary disease or chest wall disorders. Arterial oxygen saturation, ventilation and effects on inspiratory muscle effort were monitored. Results showed no clinically significant differences between the volume-present flow generator and inspiratory pressure support. Compared to spontaneous ventilation, inspiratory muscle effort decreased, tidal volume increased and respiratory frequency was reduced to a similar degree with the volume-preset flow generator and inspiratory pressure support system, but only the volume-preset system increased minute ventilation (Figs 3.1, 3.2). During CPAP, ventilation was unchanged, but inspiratory muscle effort fell by a lesser degree

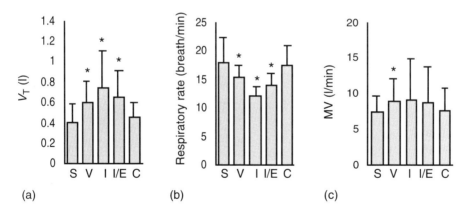

Fig. 3.1 Comparison of the effects of different modes of NIPPV and continuous positive airway pressure on mean (s.d.) (a) tidal volume, (b) respiratory rate and (c) minute volume for spontaneous ventilation (S), NIPPV with volume cycled flow generator (V), inspiratory positive airway pressure with (I/E) and without (I) expiratory airflow and continuous positive airway pressure (C). $*P < 0.05$ (compared to S). (Reproduced with permission from Elliott *et al.* [1]).

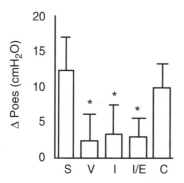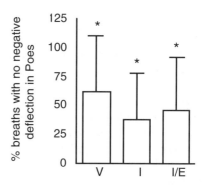

Fig. 3.2 Mean (s.d.) change in oesophageal pressure (Poes) and inspiratory muscle effort for spontaneous ventilation (S), NIPPV with volume cycled flow generator (V), inspiratory positive airway pressure with (I/E) and without (I) expiratory positive airway pressure and continuous positve airway pressure (C). *$P < 0.05$ (compared to S). (Reproduced with permission from Elliott *et al.* [1]).

(Fig. 3.2). Importantly, arterial oxygen saturation was increased by all ventilation modes, but was worse using CPAP than during spontaneous ventilation. The study was carried out in awake stable subjects who were acclimatized to ventilatory assistance. Clearly, the actions of these systems may vary during sleep (see below).

In another study [2] of stable patients, two volume-preset and two pressure-preset nasal ventilators (BromptonPAC, Monnal D, BiPAP and Nippy) were compared. Arterial blood gases were measured before and after 2 hours of NIPPV using each ventilator in random order in eight acclimatized patients with either COPD or thoracoplasty. All assessments were carried out during the day while the subjects were awake. No significant differences in PaO_2 and $PaCO_2$ were seen with each ventilator. Visual analogue scales of patient acceptability and side-effects were similar with all machines, although there were individual variations in patient acceptability.

As breathing during sleep and wakefulness differs (Chapter 2), and most ventilators are used predominantly at night, the examination of ventilatory efficiency during sleep is especially relevant. Several such comparative

studies have been carried out. The first consists of a crossover study of volume-preset equipment versus the BiPAP ventilator used in spontaneous/timed mode (i.e. with back-up controlled ventilation in the event of apnoeic periods or profound hypoventilation) [3]. Nine stable subjects receiving NIPPV for a range of pulmonary pathologies (early onset scoliosis, paralytic scoliosis, COPD) underwent polysomnography using their standard volume-preset system, followed by repeat polysomnography 7–14 days later after familiarization with the BiPAP system. In individuals requiring an inflation pressure of more than $25\,cmH_2O$, nocturnal arterial oxygen saturation and transcutaneous PCO_2 were less well controlled using the BiPAP machine, whereas in subjects needing an inflation pressure below $25\,cmH_2O$ nocturnal oxygenation was similar or improved on BiPAP compared to the volume-preset system. This suggests that some patients requiring high inflation pressures (greater than the maximum level of $22\,cmH_2O$ generated by the standard BiPAP machine) may be better served by the generally more powerful volume-preset systems, or a pressure-preset machine that can develop higher inflation pressures. These individuals are likely to have low chest wall/lung compliance or severe airflow obstruction.

The interesting finding that the BiPAP ventilator improved nocturnal arterial oxygen saturation overnight in some patients with low inflation pressures, raised the possibility the addition of EPAP was crucial and might act to increase functional residual capacity, reduce atelectasis and potentially offset the increased work of breathing associated with intrinsic PEEP. A further trial was therefore undertaken to examine the effects of expiratory positive airway pressure [4]. Fifteen patients were studied with polysomnography using IPAP on one night and IPAP/EPAP combination on another night, in random order. Seven patients had neuromusculoskeletal disorders, 8 had COPD. IPAP was set at near maximum (mean 19.4 cmH$_2$O). End expiratory oesophageal pressure (EEPoes) was measured in 12 of the 15 subjects and EPAP level matched to EEPoes value. In subjects with no significant EEPoes, EPAP was set at 5 cmH$_2$O. Nocturnal mean minimum arterial oxygen saturation and maximum transcutaneous PCO$_2$ improved on the IPAP/EPAP combination compared to IPAP alone in the neuromusculoskeletal group. Overall there was no change between the IPAP and IPAP/EPAP nights in the COPD group, although 3 of 8 patients did show an improvement in minimum SaO$_2$ or maximum TcCO$_2$ or both with the application of EPAP. All patients receiving an EPAP of 5 cmH$_2$O (n = 10) demonstrated benefit, whereas the 5 subjects receiving higher levels of EPAP (6–12 cmH$_2$O) showed no significant change. The results indicate that EPAP can be helpful in patients with neuromusculoskeletal disorders and in selected patients with COPD (Figs 3.3 and 3.4). High levels of EPAP (>5 cmH$_2$O) appear to offset any beneficial effects on functional residual capacity by either increasing expiratory muscle load

and/or reducing effective IPAP, especially in patients with severe airflow obstruction. An additional concern is that the application of EPAP could result in haemodynamic compromise. Ambrosino *et al.* [5] measured pulmonary artery wedge pressure and cardiac output in stable severe chronic COPD patients receiving IPAP and IPAP/EPAP over a 10-minute period. When compared to baseline values pulmonary wedge pressure rose and cardiac output and oxygen delivery fell with the addition of EPAP. The changes were small and it is difficult to know whether adaptive mechanisms would come into play when an IPAP/EPAP combination is used over a longer period, e.g. all night. A reasonable approach would be to use low levels of EPAP and monitor carefully the respiratory and haemodynamic response. EPAP should also be used with caution in patients with bullous lung disease and other risk factors for a pneumothorax.

TRIGGERED/ASSIST-CONTROL OR CONTROLLED VENTILATION?

Ventilators can operate in an assist mode, assist-control (A/C), or control mode. In assist mode the user is required to trigger each breath, whereas in assist-control mode breaths can be triggered, but there is a back-up controlled automatic cycling rate if the patient can no longer trigger the machine. In control mode ventilation is delivered regardless of the patient's respiratory effort. Many authorities believe that in conscious subjects, breathing is most comfortably and safely augmented by an assist/control pattern. Certainly in some patients with neuromuscular disorders, scoliosis and central hypoventilation a back-up controlled rate is often necessary to deal with apnoeic episodes, or profound hypoventilation during REM sleep (Fig. 3.5). Controlled ventilation is advocated by some workers [6] to maximally

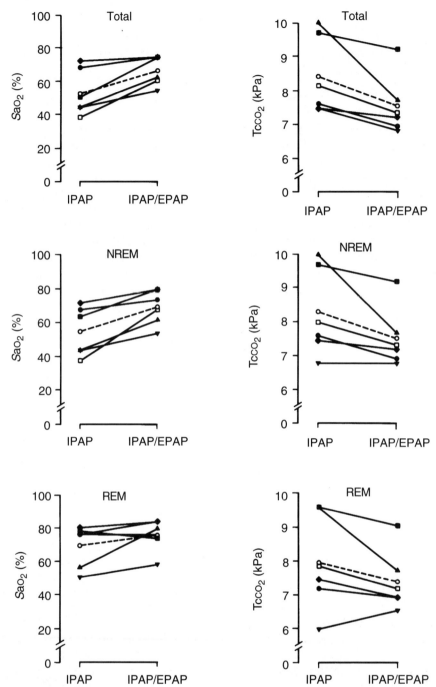

Fig. 3.3 Comparison of the effect of IPAP alone and IPAP/EPAP on minimum SaO_2 and maximum $TcCO_2$ during total sleep time (Total), NREM sleep and REM sleep in patients with restrictive chest wall disease. Dotted lines represent mean values.

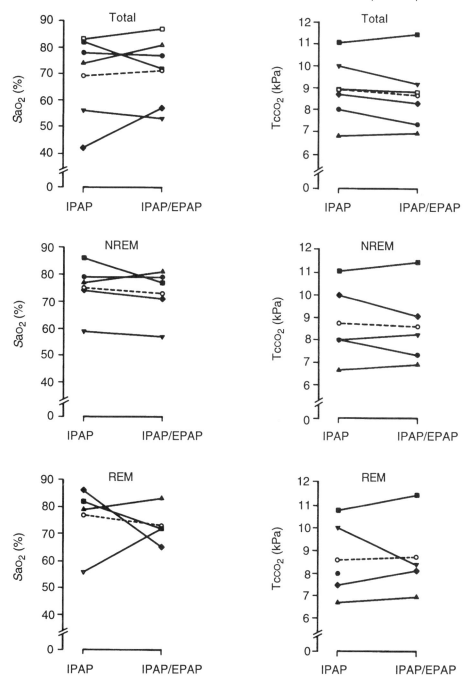

Fig. 3.4 Comparison of the effect of IPAP alone and IPAP/EPAP on minimum Sao_2 and maximum $Tcco_2$ during total sleep time (Total), NREM sleep and REM sleep in patients with chronic obstructive pulmonary disease. Dotted lines represent mean values.

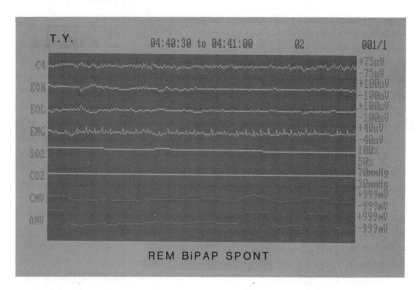

T.Y.   04:40:30 to 04:41:00   02   001/1

REM BiPAP SPONT

Fig. 3.5 Failure of triggering during REM sleep in patient using BiPAP ventilator in spontaneous (triggered) mode. CMV = chest wall movement, AMU = abdominal movement.

reduce the work of breathing and rest the respiratory muscles. There are disadvantages to this approach in that patients can become desynchronized from the imposed respiratory rate and overventilation is a distinct possibility, especially in neuromuscular patients with low minute ventilation requirements. The ensuing rapid fall in Pa_{CO_2} can provoke dysrhythmias [7], vasoconstriction and cerebral hypoperfusion. Active glottic closure may occur as a protective mechanism in this situation [8]. A common finding is that although patients use the triggered mode while awake, as Pa_{CO_2} falls ventilation is effectively 'captured' so that respiratory effort on the part of the patient during sleep is minimal. This reduction in workload may be of benefit to the respiratory muscles.

TRIGGER CHARACTERISTICS

The performance of the trigger is a key factor. Inspiratory work is decreased by a sensitive trigger with a short response time. A brief refractory period after activation of inspiration is helpful to prevent 'breath stacking' in response to frequent ineffectual ventilatory efforts. This is particularly relevant in COPD patients in whom poor coordination with the ventilator has been demonstrated. The problem can be minimized by altering the trigger sensitivity.

COMMONLY USED VOLUME-PRESET NASAL VENTILATORS

See Appendix A for details of manufacturers.

Lifecare PLV-100 (Fig. 3.6)

This volume-cycled flow generator is relatively portable and has the advantage of an internal battery and facilities for operating via an external battery. This may be particularly useful in patients who travel extensively or who need ventilatory assistance in a wheelchair. The PLV-100 can also be used to transport ventilator-dependent individuals. An internal 12 V DC battery provides continuous use for approximately 1 hour.

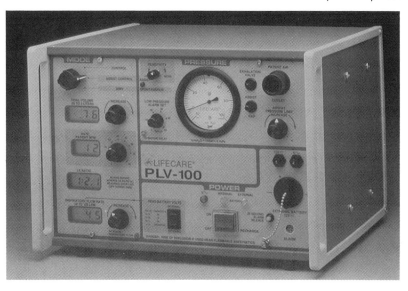

Fig. 3.6 Lifecare PLV-100 ventilator. (Courtesy of Lifecare).

The PLV-100 can be operated in assist-control, controlled, or synchronized intermittent mandatory (SIMV) mode. Tidal volume, inspiratory flow rate and a back-up respiratory rate need to be set for each patient. The ventilator calculates and displays a inspiratory:expiratory time ratio from the tidal volume, inspiratory flow rate and breaths per minute settings. Inspiratory flow rate can be adjusted from 10 to 120 litres per minute, so that if flow rate is increased without changing volume and breaths per minute, expiratory time will increase. Flow rate can be decreased to reduce peak inflation pressure. Airway pressure is displayed on the front panel (range −10 to 100 cmH$_2$O). Tidal volume can be widely adjusted from 0.05 to 3 litres, making the machine versatile and capable of ventilating both children and adults with a wide range of ventilatory requirements. Made in the United States, it is, however, more expensive than many UK and European models (cost approximately £6000). Its reliability record is good, with most models having a working life of more than seven years. Servicing is required twice a year. The PLV-100 has audible low pressure, high pressure, apnoea, ventilator malfunction, low battery and power failure alarms. A 3 second alarm sounds when the ventilator switches from mains power to internal or external battery power to alert the user that limited operation time remains.

Dimensions are: 22.9 cm high × 31.1 wide × 31.1 cm deep; weight 12.8 kg. US models operate on a 120 V AC 50/60 Hz power source; foreign models for European use employ the usual 220/240 V AC 50/60 Hz power source. There is no 220 V AC/120 V AC dual voltage model.

Monnal D/DCC (Fig. 3.7)

The Monnal D is a basic volume-preset flow generator which functions in assist-control mode. It has no internal or external battery facility. It is generally reliable, and has been developed and used extensively in France. Flow rate can be varied up to 20 litres per minute. Back-up respiratory rate, trigger sen-

23

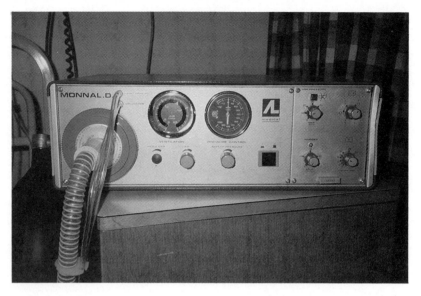

Fig. 3.7 Monnal D ventilator.

sitivity and I:E ratio need to be preset. Inflation pressure is displayed. A black rubber airbag at the side of the machine demonstrates inspiratory and expiratory activity allowing flow rate to be tailored to the patient's needs. There is no refractory period programmed into the trigger so that breath stacking may occur. The maximum flow rate of 20 litres per minute means that the machine may not be suitable for patients with high ventilatory requirements.

Dimensions are: 16 cm high × 47 cm wide × 31 cm deep; weight 14 kg.

The Monnal DCC is a newer, more versatile model. In addition to the features in the Monnal D, it has an internal battery, can be powered by an external battery source, and has an optional oxygen analyser and sigh mode. The expiratory limb of the circuit is separate from the inspiratory limb, making the equipment more bulky. Positive end expiratory pressure can be added.

Dimensions are: 22 cm high × 39 cm wide × 41 cm deep; weight 22 kg.

The Monnal D costs approximately £3800

and the DCC £5100. There is no 120 V AC version.

PneuPAC BromptonPAC (Fig. 3.8)

This time-cycled flow generator was specifically designed in the UK for nasal ventilation in the home. It has subsequently been used widely in hospitals for patients with acute respiratory failure. The ventilator comprises two parts – a compressor (AirPAC) and control module (BromptonPAC). Controls have been simplified for ease of use by patients and staff. Design specifications include A/C mode with sensitive trigger which includes a refractory period, and a high ventilatory capacity to cope with individuals with increased thoracic impedance due to either low chest wall/pulmonary compliance or high airways resistance. Flow rate can be set between 0.7 and 1.3 litres per second, with independent control of inspiratory time (TI) and expiratory time (TE). High flow rates are required to compensate for leaks from the mouth and around the mask, and to over-

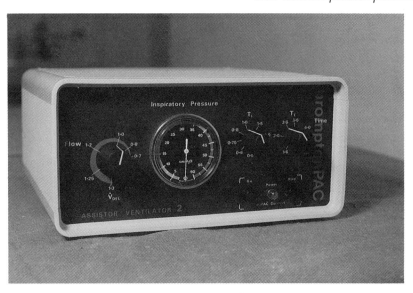

Fig. 3.8 PneuPAC BromptonPAC control module showing flow, inspiratory time (TI), expiratory time (TE) controls and inspiratory pressure gauge.

come the inefficiency of added upper airway deadspace. For adults with low ventilatory needs, and in children the PneuPAC machine may be too powerful, resulting in a rapid fall in P_{CO_2}. When spontaneous triggering occurs, TE is determined by the patient. In the absence of any ventilatory effort from the user the ventilator cycles to inspiration after the preset expiratory time, so that back-up controlled ventilation is provided. A 'hold' knob on the front of the control module allows placement of the mask before starting ventilation. Airway pressure is displayed. The compressor is mains operated and connected to the control module via an airline and electrical supply to power the high pressure, low pressure and electrical disconnection alarms. There is no battery option. Expiration is via a modified Bennett capsule valve. Early versions of the AirPAC with 12 V DC motor were unreliable, requiring frequent brush changes. Reliability has been good since substitution of a 240 V AC motor in all current models (Medical Devices Directorate

Evaluation, Department of Health, 1993). The ventilator requires servicing every six months.

For use with a compressed air outlet (e.g. in an intensive care unit or high dependency unit) the control module can be operated via an AdaptorPAC. The BromptonPAC also can be powered by a standard oxygen cylinder using a TransPAC connector. Air entrainment with this system produces an inspired oxygen concentration of around 30%. This combination can be used to transport ventilator-dependent patients. Both the AdaptorPAC and TransPAC are available fron PneuPAC Ltd.

Dimensions are: BromptonPAC, 11 cm high × 24 cm wide × 25 cm deep; weight 3.6 kg; AirPAC, 40.5 cm high × 46 cm wide × 26 cm deep; weight 17 kg. Noise emission of the AirPAC is 55 dbA at a distance of 1 metre in a laboratory environment (i.e. no carpet on floor or soft furnishings to absorb sound). The cost of the AirPAC and BromptonPAC system is around £3000. The AdaptorPAC is £580.

Companion 2801 (Puritan Bennett)

The Companion 2801 is a US-designed volume-cycled ventilator. Like the PLV-100, it operates in A/C, control or SIMV mode. It has an internal battery and can be powered by an external battery. Flow rate, volume and breathing rate (BPM) are preset. There is an additional sigh facility.

Dimensions are: 27 cm high × 32 cm wide × 34 cm deep; weight 16 kg.

COMMONLY USED PRESSURE-PRESET NASAL VENTILATORS

BiPAP (Respironics) (Fig. 3.9)

The BiPAP is a pressure-preset, pressure-limited flow generator which was orignally developed in the United States for patients with obstructive sleep apnoea/hypopnoea syndrome. Its potential for providing assisted ventilation in patients with COPD and restrictive disorders quickly became apparent. The BiPAP machine is robust and portable. Three models are produced – the BiPAP S, BiPAP S/T and BiPAP S/TD. The BiPAP S is less expensive than the other models and provides triggered ventilation only, with no back-up control mode. This makes it unsuitable for patients with depressed ventilatory drive or marked hypoventilation/central apnoea during sleep. The BiPAP S/T can function in triggered 'S' mode, assist-control 'S/T' mode or control 'T' mode. The S/TD model provides output signals of estimated tidal volume, flow rate and pressure that can be interfaced with a recorder or oscilloscope. All models can provide continuous positive airway pressure (CPAP). In each ventilatory mode a pressure support pattern of ventilation is generated. Inspiratory positive pressure and expiratory positive pressure need to be set and a back-up respiratory rate (BPM) if the S/T machine is used. In T (timed) mode the percentage of time in inspiration can be varied. With a maximum inspiratory positive pressure level of around 20 cmH$_2$O, the BiPAP machine may not be powerful enough for patients with low chest wall and pulmonary compliance (see above). In these circumstances a pressure-preset machine with higher pressure capacity (e.g. Nippy) or

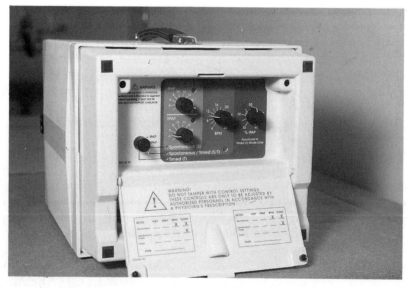

Fig. 3.9 BiPAP ventilator (Respironics Inc.).

volume-preset ventilator should be considered. A higher pressure BiPAP model will soon be available. Expiratory positive pressure may be useful in the circumstances outlined above. Expiration occurs via a 'whisper' swivel valve which connects to the mask. As the BiPAP machine is not intended for life support, the standard system does not incorporate any alarms. Each model has a voltage selector switch which allows operation at 115 and 230 V. This is valuable in patients travelling to the USA. It is important to provide a suitable fuse when the voltage is changed. The BiPAP has no internal battery and cannot be operated by external battery. The BiPAP S/T model costs approximately £4000. The S model is slightly less expensive. A higher pressure BiPAP ventilator (to 30 cm H_2O) has recently been introduced.

Dimensions are: 23 cm high × 20 cm wide × 31 cm deep; weight 4 kg.

Nippy (Thomas Respiratory Systems)
(Fig. 3.10)

The Nippy is a portable pressure-preset ventilator which can provide a maximum output pressure of 35 cm H_2O. Versions delivering higher pressures (up to 50 cm H_2O) can be ordered individually from the manufacturer. A/C ventilation is delivered, with a facility to alter trigger sensitivity. Inspiratory pressure, inspiratory time and expiratory time need to be preset. High and low pressure alarms are fitted. The machine is quiet in operation.

Dimensions are: height 26 cm × length 37 cm × depth 23 cm; weight 7.3 kg. Cost per unit is £3900, but the price is reduced for bulk purchases.

DP90 (Taema – UK suppliers Deva Medical)
(Fig. 3.11)

The DP90 is a bi-level pressure support system offering IPAP/EPAP or CPAP mode. A PEEP or EPAP level is set with the pressure difference indicating IPAP level. Maximum pressure difference is 15 cm H_2O. Respiratory frequency of 6–25 breaths per minute can be set in bi-level mode. Pressure is displayed as a liquid crystal bar chart on the front of the machine. The DP90 is one of the smallest

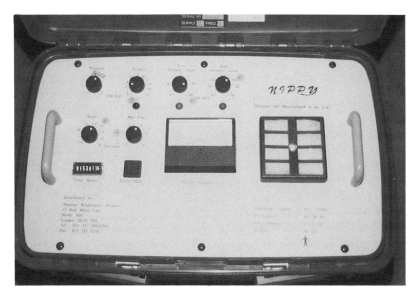

Fig. 3.10 Nippy ventilator (Thomas Respiratory Systems).

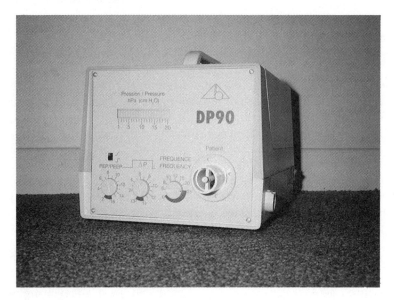

Fig. 3.11 DP90 bi-level pressure ventilator (Taema).

ventilators available (17 × 14 × 23 cm) and is lightweight at 2.9 kg. A humidifier assembly, VP90 alarm module and DC 12–24 V kit are available separately from the manufacturers. Cost is around £2550.

✴ SELECTING A VENTILATOR

If patients with a variety of respiratory pathologies are managed in a unit, a range of ventilators may be required to suit all needs. However, diversification into a wide range of ventilators is not advisable as staff will take longer to become familiar with the equipment and replacement models and parts will be more difficult to obtain. In the author's unit at the Royal Brompton Hospital we currently use a combination of PneuPAC, BiPAP, DP90 and Nippy machines, but in the past have used PLV-100 and Monnal D ventilators.

✣ PATIENT INTERFACE

Non-invasive positive pressure ventilation can be delivered via nasal mask, nasal pillows, nasal seals, full facemask (Fig. 3.12) or mouthpiece. Particular care needs to be taken when choosing and fitting the patient interface to avoid trauma to the bridge of the nose and to ensure patient comfort (see Chapter 4). If the patient is unhappy with the mask or facepiece, the system will be poorly tolerated and the attempts at assisted ventilation are likely to fail.

✣ NASAL MASKS (Fig. 3.12)

Commercial masks are obtainable from Respironics Inc., Rescare UK and Healthdyne Technologies. Most are made of silicone or vinyl and come in a range of sizes. A small size nasal mask suits most adult females of average build and adolescents; males tend to need a medium size mask. Nasal templates are available as a guide to the exact size required. Petite size (Respironics) is suitable for children and very small adults. Rescare make a miniature mask which is small enough to use for a newborn child. Respironics masks have a comfort flap lining the mask which reduces pressure directly on the face. The innovative bubble mask (Rescare) is parti-

28

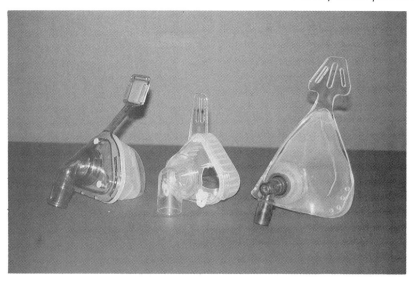

Fig. 3.12 From left: Sullivan Bubble mask, Contour silicone mask (Respironics Inc.) and full facemask (Thomas Respiratory Systems).

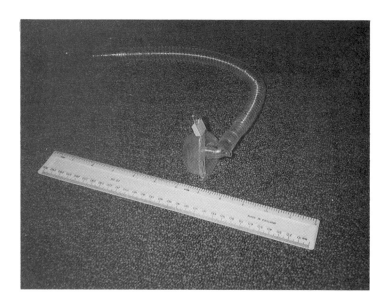

Fig. 3.13 Infant bubble mask (Rescare Ltd).

cularly useful in this respect in that the mask seals effectively by inflation of the bubble lining during inspiration, with a relaxation in pressure on the face when an airtight seal is no longer needed during expiration. Bubble masks can sometimes help heal pressure sores caused by other masks. Versions for use in infants of less than one year of age are obtainable (Fig. 3.13). Lining of the mask with towelling may help reduce leaks and

29

improve comfort in some individuals (see Chapter 14, Fig. 14.4).

NASAL PLUGS (Fig. 3.14)

Nasal plugs are a more compact form of interface which fit snugly into the nares. At least two types are manufactured: nasal pillows (Puritan Bennett) and nasal seals (Healthdyne Technologies) (Fig. 3.15). Nasal pillows are available in three sizes. Patients often find nasal plugs less claustrophobic than a mask. Occasionally they may slip from the nose during the night, but the fit is usually secure in relatively immobile patients. As the bridge of the nose and the cheeks and lower lip are left free, the nasal plugs will aid healing of pressure sores caused by a mask, and also allow the user to wear spectacles while receiving ventilation.

CUSTOMIZED NASAL MASKS AND FACEPIECES

In France nasal ventilation was pioneered using customized masks. These can be

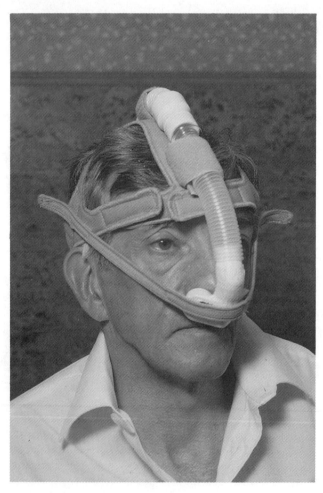

Fig. 3.14 Nasal pillows or 'plugs' (Adam circuit) (Puritan Bennett).

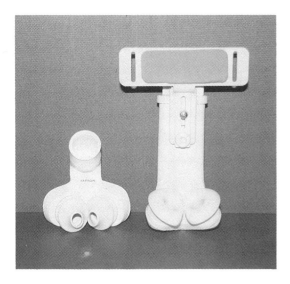

Fig. 3.15 Left nasal pillows (Puritan Bennett); *right,* nasal seals (Healthdyne Technologies).

made from kit form (e.g. Sefam kit) and are especially useful in patients who cannot be fitted comfortably with standard sized commercial masks. Most centres find these patients comprise only a small minority of those requiring ventilatory assistance and customized masks are, of course, essential for subjects requiring emergency ventilation. However, some units continue to provide customized masks for all elective patients. These masks may be less costly than commercial masks, but unless well constructed they do not always last as well. Dental appliance departments can be helpful in providing expertise and materials for facial moulds.

FACEMASKS (RESPIRONICS, THOMAS RS) (Fig. 3.12)

Full facemasks are indicated in the following situations.

1. Patient too confused to understand advice to breathe through nose.

2. Mouth leak which is not reduced by chin strap.
3. For ventilating children and infants.
4. Nasal pathology.
5. Patient preference.

Facemasks reduce the ability of the patients to communicate with carers and may lead to an increase in gastric distension. Theoretically there is a risk of aspiration of gastric contents, but we have not found this to be a problem in practice. The Respironics facemask is provided with a quick release strap to use if vomiting or aspiration occur.

The full facemask may be valuable during the first night of ventilation in patients started electively or acutely on NIPPV. In this situation REM rebound is common causing long periods of reduction in jaw tone and a marked mouth leak. A soft cervical collar will help extend the neck and improve airway patency in this situation. These measures can usually be discontinued after 24–48 hours of effective ventilation.

HEADGEAR

Masks and nasal pillows or seals are held in place with soft elasticated headgear either in the form of strapping or a cap. The mask is attached to the headgear by adjustable Velcro strips. Headgear is almost always available from the company supplying the mask or interface and is often specific for different types of mask. Chin straps can be used at night to reduce mouth leak; these also attach to the headgear via Velcro pads. Headgear and mask combinations are available to direct the tubing downwards and sideways to the bedside or upwards over the head (Fig. 3.16).

PATIENT MAINTENANCE OF EQUIPMENT

It is recommended that masks and tubing are washed in soapy water once a week. Sterilization is not required and should be avoided as chemicals will damage the mask and

31

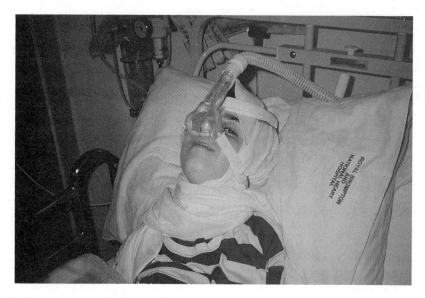

Fig. 3.16 Nasal mask (Healthdyne Technologies) with over the head tubing.

tubing. Headgear and chinstraps should be washed on a regular basis. Filters on some ventilators require replacement or washing. The synthetic filters on the BromptonPAC and compressor should be washed weekly and dried before replacing. Disposable filters on the BiPAP need replacing approximately every few weeks.

MOUTHPIECE VENTILATION

Mouthpiece ventilation has a number of advocates and is used extensively in several centres in the USA and France. Bach [9] has reported the use of MIPPV as an alternative to tracheostomy in 257 patients. The majority of patients had neuromuscular disorders (mainly previous poliomyelitis) and used MIPPV at night. Sixty-one had little or no measurable vital capacity and were almost entirely ventilator-dependent. All motivated patients with sufficient oropharyngeal strength to swallow and speak intelligibly were able to use MIPPV effectively. Lip seal retention devices were used to secure the

mouthpiece at night. A strapless oral interface (SONI) has also been devised [10,11]. Complications of MIPPV include orthodontic deformity, leaks from the nose and air swallowing. Despite the lipseal, three patients in the Newark series [9] died during sleep following accidental disconnection from the ventilator. MIPPV can be particularly helpful as an adjunct during the day for wheelchair-bound individuals.

NEGATIVE PRESSURE VENTILATION

TANK VENTILATOR OR IRON LUNG

The basic design of the tank ventilator has changed little since Drinker's original model (Chapter 1). The machines are large and bulky, as the whole of the trunk of the individual from the neck down is enclosed. A sizeable pump is required to generate a negative pressure of up to $40\,cmH_2O$ in the chamber. The pump may be incorporated in the base of the machine or freestanding. Simple early versions employ a variable leak

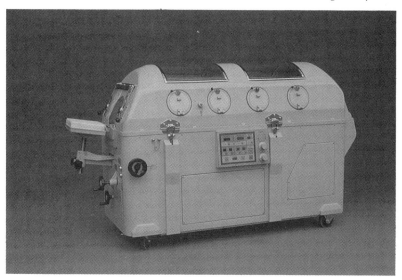

Fig. 3.17 Iron lung. (Courtesy of Coppo Biella).

to adjust pressure and fixed inspiratory rate. Recent models incorporate a programmable rate, pressure setting and I:E ratio (Fig. 3.17). Lightweight Perspex or fibreglass versions that can be used in the home (e.g. Portalung) have also been developed. Around 100 patients still use iron lungs on a long-term basis in the UK and negative pressure systems are widely used in Italy and in some centres in the USA.

CUIRASS

The cuirass shell is an alternative, albeit less efficient method of delivering negative pressure ventilation. The shell is made of plastic or vithrane and fits over the anterior and lateral chest wall, being held in place by a strap encircling the trunk. Ventilation is less effective than using the iron lung as a smaller area of chest wall is enclosed and chest expansion is limited at the rim of the cuirass. A cuirass needs to be individually contructed for patients with chest wall deformity and this expertise is not widely available. A

further disadvantage is that the equipment works best in the supine position with troublesome leaks occurring if the patient sits up or turns on to one side.

Chest wall irritation and pressure sores sometimes occur if the cuirass is not well fitted. An important advantage of the cuirass is that it requires minimal manual dexterity to put on, so may be indicated in disabled individuals with weakness of the upper limbs. Pumps suitable for evacuating a cuirass are the Siplan pump, Emerson negative pressure ventilator and Lifecare NEV-100 system (see Appendix A).

PNEUMOJACKET/SUIT/PONCHO (Fig. 3.18)

This system consists of a airtight nylon garment which fits over a frame covering the chest wall. The garment is sealed beneath the frame with a belt and secured with ties around the arms. As a larger area of chest wall is enclosed than with the cuirass, the pneumosuit system tends to be more mech-

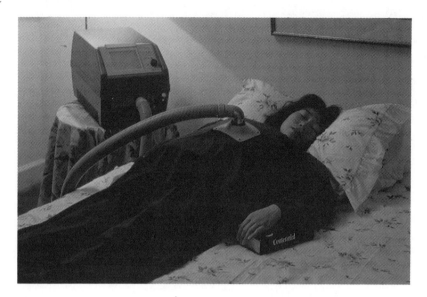

Fig. 3.18 Pneumosuit.

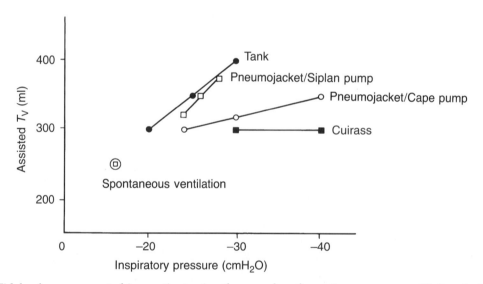

Fig. 3.19 Tidal volumes generated in a patient using three modes of negative pressure ventilation: tank ventilaor (iron lung), pneumosuit system and cuirass.

anically efficient than the cuirass, but less effective than the iron lung (Fig. 3.19). The jackets and frames are simpler to make than a cuirass. Commercial jackets and frames are available from the manufacturers listed in Appendix A. The Siplan, Emerson and Lifecare NEV-100 negative pressure ventilators can be used. As with the cuirass, the

34

pneumojacket needs to be worn in the supine position and can cause backache. Some patients find the pneumojacket difficult to assemble and put on without assistance. Negative pressures of between 15 and 30 cmH$_2$O are usually required.

HAYEK OSCILLATOR (Fig. 3.20)

The Hayek Oscillator is a modification of the cuirass in which an oscillating level of pressure is superimposed on to a negative pressure baseline. This form of ventilatory support is termed external high frequency oscillation (EHFO). Pressures of up to -100 cmH$_2$O can be generated with an oscillation frequency of up to 999 cycles/minute. In practice lower oscillation pressures are better tolerated initially (30–90/minute) and little improvement in CO$_2$ clearance is seen above 180/minute. I:E ratio may be varied, and there are 12 sizes of cuirass shell available. The Hayek Oscillator can be used in adults and children. There are two power units – an adult model with maximum stroke volume of

4 litres and paediatric version with stroke volume of 1.45 litres.

NEGATIVE VERSUS POSITIVE PRESSURE VENTILATION

The advantages and disadvantages of non-invasive negative pressure systems are outlined below.

Advantages
• Can be used in all age groups, including infants.
• Some devices (e.g. cuirass) require minimal dexterity to apply.
• May be used in patients with nasal airway obstruction.
• Can add high frequency oscillation.

Disadvantages
• Equipment bulky.
• Expertise with NPV limited to small number of centres in some countries.
• Can predispose to upper airway obstruction.
• Negative pressure pumps are often fixed rate as it is difficult to develop triggered systems.
• Reduced mechanical efficiency compared to NIPPV.
• Can provoke back pain and claustrophobia.

VENTILATORY ADJUNCTS

THE ROCKING BED

The rocking bed employs gravity-assisted movement of the abdominal contents to facilitate diaphragm excursion. As a consequence it can be used in individuals with bilateral diaphragm weakness. However, the augmentation in tidal volume is often minor and patient mobility is limited. The rocking bed is inappropriate in patients with poor control of the airway and in patients with more than modest ventilatory needs, particularly those with chest wall deformity and

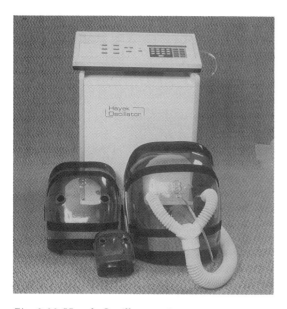

Fig. 3.20 Hayek Oscillator cuirass system.

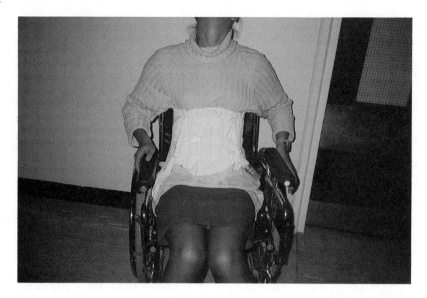

Fig. 3.21 Pneumobelt.

chronic airflow obtruction. Goldstein *et al.* [12] compared the rocking bed with cuirass nPV and showed a greater fall in Pa_{CO_2} and respiratory muscle activity using nPV. Interestingly, motion sickness is not a problem with the rocking bed, as it rotates through a single plane.

PNEUMOBELT (Fig. 3.21)

The pneumobelt consists of an expandable rubber bladder contained within an abdominal corset. Inflation of the bladder to around $+50\,cmH_2O$ causes active expiration by abdominal displacement. This system can be used in a wheelchair-bound patient and may act as an adjunct to other ventilatory methods such as NIPPV. We have found it useful for daytime 'top-up' respiratory support in some individuals with Duchenne muscular dystrophy. The pneumobelt works more effectively with the patient sitting upright, but may interfere with nasogastric feeding and precludes the use of a gastrostomy. Positive pressure ventilators such as the high pressure version of the Nippy

(Thomas Respiratory Systems) will power the pneumobelt. The cost of the pneumobelt, which is made in several sizes, is approximately £500. Dougherty [13] has devised a modified pneumobelt constructed of two large thigh blood pressure cuffs and inflated by an Aequitron LP6 volume-preset ventilator.

REFERENCES

1. Elliott, M.W., Aquilina, R., Green, M. *et al.* (1994) A comparison of different modes of non-invasive ventilatory support: effects on ventilation and inspiratory muscle effort. *Anaesthesia*, **49**, 279–283.
2. Meecham Jones, D.J., Braid, G. and Wedzicha, J.A. (1992) Nasal intermittent positive pressure ventilation: assessment and comparison of volume and pressure preset ventilator systems in chronic respiratory failure. *Thorax*, **47**, 859.
3. Simonds, A.K. and Elliott, M.W. (1991) Use of the BIPAP ventilator for non-invasive ventilation: advantages and limitations. *Am. Rev. Respir. Dis.*, **143**(Suppl.), A585.
4. Elliott, M.W. and Simonds, A.K. (1994) Nocturnal assisted ventilation using Bi-level positive airway pressure: the effect of ex-

piratory positive airway pressure. *Eur. Respir. J.*, **8**, 436–40.

5. Ambrosino, N., Nava, S., Torbicki, A. *et al.*, (1993) Haemodynamic effects of pressure support and PEEP ventilation by nasal route in patients with stable chronic obstructive pulmonary disease. *Thorax*, **48**, 523–8.

6. Rodenstein, D.O. (1992) Assist or control ventilation in nasal intermittent positive pressure ventilation. *Eur. Respir. Rev.*, **2**, 432–3.

7. Piper, A.J. and Sullivan, C.E. (1994) Breathing and neuromuscular disease, in *Sleep and Breathing* (eds N.A. Saunders and C.E. Sullivan), Marcel Dekker, New York, p. 777.

8. Delguste, P., Aubert-Tulkens, G. and Rodenstein, D.O. (1991) Upper airway obstruction during nasal intermittent positive pressure hyperventilation in sleep. *Lancet*, **338**, 1295–7.

9. Bach, J.R., Alba, A.S. and Saporito, L.R. (1993) Intermittent positive pressure ventilation via the mouth as an alternative to tracheostomy for 257 ventilator users. *Chest*, **103**, 174–82.

10. Bach, J.R. and McDermott, I.G. (1990) Strapless oral-nasal interface for positive-pressure ventilation. *Arch. Phys. Med. Rehabil.*, **71**, 910–13.

11. Sortor, S. (1992) Pulmonary issues in quadriplegia. *Eur. Respir. Rev.*, **2**, 330–4.

12. Goldstein, R.S., Molotiu, N, Skrastins, R., *et al.* (1987) Assisting ventilation in respiratory failure by negative pressure ventilation and by rocking bed. *Chest*, **92**, 470–4.

13. Dougherty, G., Davis, G.M., Gaul, M. and Diana, P. (1993) Pneumobelt assisted ventilation in Duchenne's muscular dystrophy. Proceedings of the 4th International Conference on home mechanical ventilation, Lyons, 1993, p. 65.

4

Non-invasive ventilation in acute respiratory failure

ANITA K. SIMONDS and MARK W. ELLIOTT

INTRODUCTION

While methods of supplying ventilatory assistance without an endotracheal tube have been associated historically with the development of domiciliary respiratory support, both negative pressure and mask ventilation techniques were used as resuscitation aids as early as the 1830s. Predating this, the Royal Humane Society's resuscitation apparatus of 1774, displayed at the Association of Anaesthetists, includes masks and connections for nasal ventilation, in addition to a set of bellows and a metal cannula which was designed for tracheal placement. This equipment was provided to houses on the banks of the Thames, and later in coastal areas in England and on the Continent.

In acute hypercapnic respiratory failure, non-invasive techniques have the advantage of simplicity and avoidance of the complications of intubation. As they can be used on a general or high dependency ward, intensive care admissions may be reduced. The majority of patients with an acute exacerbation of chronic lung disease have COPD, but there is a sizeable number of individuals with chest wall disorders and neuromuscular disease who are also liable to hypercapnic decompensation following a chest infection or surgery.

Negative pressure ventilation (nPV) has been employed in some centres extensively for patients with acute respiratory failure over the past few decades, but practical restrictions and the limited availability of equipment and expertise has meant that use of nPV has never become widespread. In contrast, NIPPV and mask ventilation are easily applied in acute situations and most staff are familiar with masks from the regular use of CPAP.

NASAL/FACEMASK VENTILATION IN ACUTE EXACERBATIONS OF COPD

There is a perception that patients with COPD who are intubated and mechanically ventilated have a poor prognosis. To some extent these problems are probably overstated, with good results reported by units who adopt an aggressive approach. In an analysis of 100 consecutive intensive care unit (ICU) admissions of patients with severe COPD (mean FEV_1 0.7 litres) of whom 32% were receiving home oxygen therapy and 42% were housebound, Moran et al. [1]

Non-Invasive Respiratory Support. Edited by Anita Simonds. Published by Chapman & Hall, London. ISBN 0412 56840 3.

reported ICU, hospital and 6-month mortality of 1.5%, 13% and 27% respectively. Despite these encouraging figures, the outcome in other series is less good [2] and there is often reluctance to admit such patients to scarce ICU facilities. The option of non-invasive ventilation offers several potential advantages. Patients retain a degree of control denied them when intubated and can participate in decisions about their management. Nutrition can be maintained orally and patients can cooperate with physiotherapy. Ventilatory support can be gradually withdrawn, first during the day and subsequently at night as well. There have been a number of descriptive studies reporting varying degrees of success. Meduri and co-workers [3] were among the first to report the use of facemask pressure support ventilation in acute respiratory failure. They treated COPD patients who fulfilled criteria for intubation and mechanical ventilation (mean pH 7.29, $Paco_2$ 9.6 kPa) and found that adequate ventilation was secured with the facemask, although 40% of patients ultimately required intubation. In a follow-up study [4] of 18 patients, facemask ventilation was successful in avoiding intubation in 13. Mean duration of ventilatory support was 25 hours. The mask was well tolerated in all but two patients. Gastric aspiration occurred in one individual and mild skin necrosis developed in another patient.

A matched historical controlled study was performed by Brochard and colleagues [5]. They used inspiratory pressure support via a full facemask for an average of 7 hours per day for between 2 and 6 days in 13 patients with an acute exacerbation who they judged would probably have needed intubation. Only one of the patients receiving facemask ventilation required intubation compared with 11 of 13 in the control group and the non-invasive ventilation group spent less time in the ICU. Mortality was similar in both groups.

Foglio *et al.* [6] carried out a retrospective controlled study of nasal ventilation using a volume-preset ventilator in 25 COPD patients with an acute hypercapnic exacerbation (mean pH 7.33, $Paco_2$ 9.8 kPa), although in this study the need for intubation was an indication for exclusion from the study. The regime used was unusual in that it consisted of NIPPV being applied for 1 hour, four times a day for 3 weeks. The improvement in arterial blood gas tensions, airflow obstruction and respiratory muscle strength was similar to the control group who received standard measures without nasal ventilation. Side-effects, mainly mask discomfort and dry nose, were seen in between 20 and 30% of patients. Compliance rates were unclear, and although the result was negative, it is difficult to see the relevance of this regime to the care of most patients admitted with an acute exacerbation.

So far only one prospective randomized controlled trial of nasal ventilation in acute COPD has been reported in detail [7]. Here volume-preset ventilation via nasal mask was compared to conventional therapy in patients with an acute hypercapnic exacerbation (mean $Paco_2$ 8.6 kPa). Thirty patients were randomized to receive NIPPV and 30 patients received conventional therapy. Non-invasive ventilation was used as intensively as tolerated in the first few days of treatment. Nasal ventilation was more effective than standard treatment in lowering $Paco_2$ and reversing acidosis (Fig. 4.1). Mortality in the conventionally treated group was 9/30 patients, and in the NIPPV group 2/30 patients. This difference does not reach statistical significance when analysed on an intention to treat basis. Four patients allocated to NIPPV did not receive this therapy: one had a chronic nose injury which made NIPPV impossible, one patient refused all treatment, and two patients, one of whom died, were confused and unable to cooperate. A treatment efficacy comparison of the 26 patients

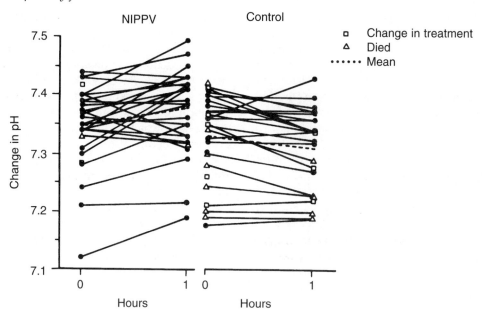

Fig. 4.1 Effect of NIPPV on arterial pH in patients with an acute exacerbation of COPD. (Reproduced with permission from Bott *et al.* [7]).

who received NIPPV and the 30 patients who received conventional therapy demonstrated a significant reduction in mortality in the NIPPV group ($P = 0.01$). It should be noted that NIPPV was not feasible in 13% of COPD patients.

Nasal ventilation has been compared with the ventilatory stimulant doxapram in COPD patients with acute respiratory failure [8]. Similar groups were randomized to either doxapram or pressure-preset NIPPV. After 4 hours, arterial blood tensions improved in the NIPPV group, but $Paco_2$ was unchanged in the patients receiving doxapram. At 24 hours three out of five patients had died in doxapram group, and therefore the protocol was modified such that any patient still deteriorating at 4 hours was switched to the other limb of the study. Subsequently two patients were switched to NIPPV, but none from NIPPV to doxapram. The two individuals who were changed from doxapram to NIPPV showed improvements

in Pao_2 and $Paco_2$ suggesting that NIPPV may be more effective and safer than doxapram, although the study contained only 11 patients and results are preliminary.

Information from a number of studies suggest that the factors most likely to predict success from NIPPV in acute respiratory failure are an early fall in $Paco_2$ and rise in pH. This is not surprising as arterial hydrogen ion concentration is a consistent prognostic factor in exacerbations of COPD [2]. The long-term outcome of COPD patients who are treated acutely with NIPPV is not known. Data from one unit [9] indicate 37% mortality at one year and that 28% of patients had required a further course of NIPPV. There is no information on functional status or quality of life in this group.

The choice of ventilator does not seem to be an important determinant of success. Ambrosino *et al.* [10] showed no difference in outcome in COPD patients treated with pressure support and volume-preset ventilation, although patients were not randomized to the type of ventilation. A cross-over study of pressure support at various levels, volume-preset ventilation and CPAP in acute COPD patients has demonstrated similar effects on arterial blood gas tensions [11].

NIPPV IN ACUTE EXACERBATIONS IN RESTRICTIVE DISORDERS

Many studies concerning the use of NIPPV in acute hypercapnic respiratory failure include some patients with chest wall disorders or neuromuscular disease. Hill [12] combined the results for four studies and showed a success rate of 67%. Patients with early onset scoliosis, previous poliomyelitis and post-tuberculous lung and chest wall disease appear to do particularly well; however, a greater proportion may need long-term ventilatory assistance. As with the COPD patients, outcome after the acute period of treatment is not well documented.

NIPPV IN ELDERLY PATIENTS

Complications associated with intubation and ICU admission are more prevalent in elderly patients. Benhamou et al. [13] have shown that age is no bar to the effective use of NIPPV. In a group of 30 patients with a mean age of 76 years in whom intubation was felt contraindicated, nasal mask ventilation using a volumetric ventilator was successful in 60% of patients. The treatment was well tolerated in 23/30. Ventilatory support was used continuously for the first 12 hours and following nights, and subsequently intermittently during the day. Sixteen patients were discharged home (11 with long-term oxygen therapy and one with home ventilation).

IMPLEMENTATION OF NIPPV

While intubation and intermittent positive pressure ventilation are often assumed to be more demanding in staff time than non-invasive techniques, Chevrolet et al. [14] have reported the opposite. Using NIPPV in an ICU in six patients they found that nurses had to monitor the three patients with restrictive disorders for 41% of the duration of ventilation and the individuals with chronic obstructive lung disease for 91% of the time. NIPPV was more successful in the restrictive group than those with obstructive lung disease. Although NIPPV may be labour-intensive during the first 24 hours of treatment, other units have not found this to be a major disincentive. Inevitably there is a learning curve when any new technique in introduced and NIPPV is no exception. In some units NIPPV is applied acutely on a general ward [15] and this is certainly possible when all team members, including junior medical staff, nurses and physiotherapists, are familiar with the equipment and its implementation. Pennock et al. [16] have outlined the issues concerning the introduction of NIPPV into routine medical practice.

NEGATIVE PRESSURE VENTILATION IN ACUTE VENTILATORY FAILURE

There are numerous reports on the use of nPV in acute respiratory failure, but these usually comprise small uncontrolled series. Negative pressure ventilation (nPV) was used extensively for acute respiratory failure in the poliomyelitis epidemics before the introduction of intermittent positive pressure ventilation. This and other historical applications of nPV are described in Chapter 1. Many polio patients who have relapsed in recent years and now use NIPPV in the home owe their lives to treatment in the tank ventilator during their acute illness.

It is clear that in the situation of acute respiratory failure the tank ventilator provides more effective ventilation than the cuirass or most pneumojacket (ponchowrap) systems, but it also restricts movement

41

and access to the patient. The newer tank ventilators (e.g. Mod. C 900, Coppa Biella) offer a greater flexibility in ventilatory settings than previous models. This flexibility may be valuable, especially in COPD patients who tend to have more complex ventilatory needs than neuromuscular patients.

In recent years Corrado *et al.* [17] have used tank ventilation in nine COPD patients with acute respiratory failure and compared results with seven controls who received similar measures other than nPV. There was a significant increase in pH, arterial blood gas tensions and mouth pressures in the nPV group, but this was not a randomized study. The same authors [18] have examined the short- and long-term effects of a course of nPV used during an acute exacerbation in 105 COPD patients. Eleven per cent died in hospital and 87% were weaned from all forms of ventilatory support. Of this latter group 82% were alive at 1 year and 37% at 5 years.

Other workers have concentrated on pneumojacket, ponchowrap treatment or cuirass treatment, which undoubtedly is effective in some cases. However there is often little mention of side-effects of treatment and patient acceptability. Problems with upper airway obstruction during sleep, back pain and immobility have bedevilled trials of nPV in individuals with chronic respiratory failure and can be hardly less of a problem in acute episodes.

CONCLUSIONS

Both nPV and NIPPV can be used to treat patients with acute ventilatory failure. nPV is unlikely to become widely available and is also less easy to implement in the acute case. NIPPV is therefore the method of choice. Controlled studies support the effectiveness of NIPPV in the patients who receive it. A proportion varying between 10 and 40% will be unable to tolerate the mask, or fail to respond. NIPPV offers a useful alternative to intubation and intensive care in patients with ventilatory failure who, for whatever reason, are felt unsuitable for endotracheal intubation. In those deemed suitable for intubation, providing they fulfil appropriate criteria, NIPPV can be tried first and if it fails the patient can then the intubated, possibly with NIPPV used to help weaning – see Chapter 6. Similar results are obtained with pressure support and volume-preset ventilators. Information is needed on the long-term outcome of patients who receive NIPPV during an acute exacerbation.

REFERENCES

1. Moran, J.L., Green, J.V., Peisach, A.R. *et al.* (1993) Outcome of a hundred episodes of acute exacerbation of chronic obstructive pulmonary disease treated in intensive care. *Eur. Respir. J.*, **6**, 177s.
2. Jeffrey, A.A., Warren, P.M. and Flenley, D.C. (1992) Acute hypercapnic respiratory failure in patients with chronic obstructive lung disease: risk factors and use of guidelines for management. *Thorax*, **47**, 34–40.
3. Meduri, G.U., Conoscenti, C.C., Menashe, P. and Nair, S. (1989) Noninvasive face mask ventilation in patients with acute respiratory failure. *Chest*, **95**, 865–70.
4. Meduri, G.U., Abou-Shala, N., Fox, R.C. *et al.* (1991) Noninvasive face mask mechanical ventilation in patients with acute hypercapneic respiratory failure. *Chest*, **100**, 445–54.
5. Brochard, L., Isabey, D., Piquet, J. *et al.* (1990) Reversal of acute exacerbations of chronic obstructive lung disease by inspiratory assistance with a face mask. *N. Engl. J. Med.*, **323**, 1523–30.
6. Foglio, C., Vitacca, M., Quadri, A. *et al.* (1992) Acute exacerbations in severe COLD patients. Treatment using positive pressure ventilation by nasal mask. *Chest*, **101**, 1533–8.
7. Bott, J., Carroll, M.P., Conway, J.H. *et al.* (1993) Randomised controlled trial of nasal ventilation in acute ventilatory failure due to chronic obstructive airways disease. *Lancet*, **341**, 1555–7.

8. Ahmed, A.H., Fenwick, L., Angus, R.M. and Peacock, A.J. (1992) Nasal ventilation *v.* doxapram in the treatment of type II respiratory failure complicating chronic airflow obstruction. *Thorax*, **47**, 858.

9. Vitacca, M., Clini, E., Nava, S. *et al.* (1994) Non invasive mechanical ventilation versus endotracheal intubation in COLD patients: differences in outcome and survival. *Eur. Respir. J.*, **7**, 416s.

10. Ambrosino, N., Nava, S., Clini, E. *et al.* (1994) Non-invasive mechanical ventilation in acute respiratory failure: is it possible to predict success in COPD? *Eur. Respir. J.*, **7**, 415s.

11. Meecham Jones, D.J., Paul, E.A., Graham-Clarke, C. and Wedzicha, J.A. (1994) Nasal ventilation in acute exacerbations of chronic obstructive pulmonary disease: effect of ventilator mode on arterial blood gases. *Thorax*, **49**, 1222–4.

12. Hill, N. (1993) Noninvasive ventilation. Does it work, for whom, and how? *Am. Rev. Respir. Dis.*, **147**, 1050–5.

13. Benhamou, D., Girault, C., Faure, C. *et al.* (1992) Nasal mask ventilation in acute respiratory failure. *Chest*, **102**, 912–17.

14. Chevrolet, J.C., Jolliet, P., Abajo, B. *et al.* (1991) Nasal positive pressure ventilation in patients with acute respiratory failure. *Chest*, **100**, 775–82.

15. Conway, J.H., Hitchcock, R.A., Godfrey, R.C. and Carroll, M.P. (1993) Nasal intermittent positive pressure ventilation in acute exacerbations of chronic obstructive pulmonary disease – a preliminary study. *Respir. Med.*, **87**, 387–94.

16. Pennock, B.E., Crawshaw, L. and Kaplan, P.D. (1994) Non-invasive nasal mask ventilation for acute respiratory failure. Institution of a new therapeutic technology for routine use. *Chest*, **105**, 441–4.

17. Corrado, A., Bruscoli, G., De Paola, E. *et al.* (1990) Respiratory muscle insufficiency in acute respiratory failure of subjects with severe COPD: treatment with intermittent negative pressure ventilation. *Eur. Respir. J.*, **3**, 644–8.

18. Corrado, A., Bruscoli, G., Messori, A. *et al.* (1992) Iron lung treatment of subjects with COPD in acute respiratory failure. Evaluation of short and long term prognosis. *Chest*, **101**, 692–6.

5

Starting nasal intermittent positive pressure ventilation: practical aspects

ANITA K. SIMONDS

INTRODUCTION

As nasal mask or facemask ventilation is the technique most likely to be available to treat patients with acute or chronic ventilatory failure, the following account is given as a guide to starting mask ventilation. The key to success lies in the selection of the appropriate patient, the choice of suitable equipment and familiarity with the technique. Individuals suitable for a trial of mask ventilation should fulfil these criteria.

- Hypercapnic respiratory failure unresponsive to conventional measures.
- Normal or near normal bulbar function.
- Ability to clear bronchial secretions.
- Haemodynamic stability.
- Functioning gastrointestinal tract.
- Able to cooperate with treatment.

The guidelines below have been used to teach the introduction of NIPPV to a number of medical and ancillary staff. It is in the nature of guidelines that the advice is didactic and some of the comments may seem obvious. The use of several types of ventilator is described. For other ventilators the same basic principles apply when establishing settings on volume-preset and pressure-preset equipment.

CHECKLIST FOR NIPPV

INITIAL ASSESSMENT

First check patient suitability.

1. Is the patient hypercapnic? In the presence of normocapnia or hypocapnia NIPPV is *not* usually indicated. NIPPV is also contraindicated in patients who have bulbar insufficiency, and in those who are comatose or who cannot clear their secretions.
2. Have conventional measures been fully explored? Ensure that controlled O_2, bronchodilator and steroid therapy (if indicated) are optimized. Is conventional intubation and ventilation the treatment of choice? (For example, in patients with acute severe asthma and hypercapnia, or gross sputum retention unresponsive to physiotherapy etc.)

Next, remember that NIPPV is not a universal panacea. Consider the following.

3. What are the reversible features in this case? Assess the patient's quality of life and prognosis. Is short- or long-term benefit likely? Do the patient and family want active treatment?

Non-Invasive Respiratory Support. Edited by Anita Simonds. Published by Chapman & Hall, London. ISBN 0412 56840 3.

4. Consider what you are going to do if NIPPV fails. Would it be appropriate to proceed to intubation and conventional ventilation?

EQUIPMENT

Assuming you wish to go ahead:

5. It is advisable to assemble the ventilator and circuit and check that it works *before* taking it to the bedside. Ensure that the tubing is connected with the expiratory valve adjacent to the mask.

6. *Explain* what you are going to do, and the sensations the patient is likely to experience. If time allows, you may be able to introduce the patient to another individual using NIPPV.

7. It is helpful to start by entraining O_2 connected by tubing to a porthole in the mask if baseline Po_2 is less than 7.0 kPa, as patients are more likely to become claustrophobic using the mask if hypoxaemia is not rapidly corrected. A flow rate of 1–2 l/min is usually sufficient.

8. The fitting of the mask is crucial to the success of the technique. A small nasal mask is usually suitable for females, males need a medium (MS or MN), but try to match to the contours and size of the patient's face. Mask fitting templates are available from some manufacturers (e.g. Respironics). If the patient uses dentures it is helpful to keep these in place. Further details on masks and other interfaces are given in Chapter 3.

If the patient is confused, a full face-mask may be preferable, but they make some individuals feel claustrophobic. Make sure that the patient is lying comfortably on the bed. It is best to let him/her hold the mask firmly to their face at first. Remind them that they should breathe through their nose and keep their mouth closed, if using a nasal mask. Once the patient is happy to continue, secure the mask in place using the headgear. Time spent building the patient's confidence at this stage is well invested.

VENTILATOR SETTINGS

Now decide on the initial ventilator settings. In this you must be guided by your patient's ventilatory needs. We find it most useful to use an assist-control (A/C) pattern of ventilation (spontaneous/timed (S/T) mode on the BiPAP (Respironics) ventilator). (See Chapter 3 for discussion of assist, assist-control and controlled ventilation options.)

For the BromptonPac (volume-preset ventilator):

Start with a fairly low flow (V) setting (left-hand knob) – around 0.7–0.8 l/s. Very tachypnoeic patients will require a shorter TI (inspiratory time) and TE (expiratory time) than patients with reduced ventilatory effort (e.g. COPD blue bloaters). Remember that the patient will usually be triggering the ventilator, so they will normally determine the TE. An average TI setting is around 1.0 seconds, with a TE set at 2.5 seconds. However, respond to what the patient feels is comfortable. It is helpful to ask 'Are you getting a big enough breath?' and adjust the flow accordingly, and 'Does the breath feel long enough?' and adjust TI accordingly. If the patient feels that the breaths are coming too fast TE may be too short. A more usual reason is patient anxiety, which should respond to reassurance. Relief of dyspnoea and a reduction or abolition of accessory muscle activity are good guides that the treatment is effective. As soon as the work of breathing lessens many acute patients fall asleep. Those in whom NIPPV is started electively, often take longer to acclimatize.

Alarms: Expect an inflation pressure of $20-40\,cmH_2O$. The dial reflects the pressure in the upper airway, not necessarily that in the lung. You may be able to adjust settings to reduce a peak inflation pressure in patients at risk of pneumothorax (e.g. by reducing flow rate or increasing TI). The upper pressure alarm should be set at around $40\,cmH_2O$. This may need to be reset in the occasional patient, e.g. those with cystic fibrosis and sputum retention.

The low pressure alarm should be set at around $8-12\,cmH_2O$. In the first 24 hours of NIPPV a balance should be struck between avoiding leaks and keeping the whole ward awake with the low pressure alarm. The usual cause for the alarm going off is because the pressure is too low due to leaks from the mouth or around the mask. The ventilator will alarm if the patient keeps talking! Most patients need a chin strap to keep the mouth shut during sleep.

For the BiPAP ventilator:

Add O_2 1–2l/min as above if $PaO_2 <$ 7 kPa. Preset an inspiratory pressure (IPAP) at around $10-14\,cmH_2O$ and leave the EPAP setting at zero initially. Use the machine in spontaneous/timed (S/T) mode. Set a back-up respiratory rate of 10–12 breaths/min. S mode (assist only) may be sufficient if central drive is not depressed.

Check SaO_2 and arterial blood gas tensions (ABG) as above. Increase the inspiratory pressure setting to reduce PCO_2. Most individuals (apart from those with neuromuscular disease) will need an inspiratory pressure of $>14\,cmH_2O$. Some patients with neuromuscular disease and COPD may benefit from the addition of a low level of EPAP (up to $5\,cmH_2O$) – see Chapter 3.

For the Nippy ventilator (Thomas Respiratory Systems):

Add O_2 1–2l/min as above if $PaO_2 <$ 7 kPa. Start at a low pressure setting, e.g. C or D ($10-15\,cmH_2O$). Set an inspiratory time of approx 1 second and an expiratory time of around 2.5 seconds. Trigger sensitivity should be low (0.5 cmH_2O) to reduce the work of breathing. The high pressure alarm should be at between 30 and $40\,cmH_2O$, the low pressure alarm at around $8-12\,cmH_2O$.

Gradually increase pressure as the patient settles on the machine. Most individuals will need a pressure of >14 cmH_2O. Adjust pressure and FIO_2 according to ABG.

MONITORING

Monitor progress in *all* patients with oximetry. Aim for an SaO_2 of $>90\%$. If this is not achieved, increase O_2 flow rate and/or adjust ventilation depending on $PaCO_2$. In severely ill patients ECG monitoring and an arterial line facilitate management. The patient will need close observation and encouragement during the initial period of NIPPV to build up confidence.

Wait at least 30 minutes before checking arterial blood gas tensions with the patient on NIPPV. *Do not* expect a major change in $PaCO_2$. The aim is adequate oxygenation and a reduction in respiratory acidosis, without an uncontrolled increase in $PaCO_2$. Nasal ventilation is relatively inefficient and so blood gases should improve gradually rather than rapidly. A rise in pH and fall in $PaCO_2$ after the first hour of NIPPV are good prognostic signs. Gradually increase ventilator flow rate or inspiratory pressure to improve PCO_2 control. An increase in TI may help improve PO_2 if the patient can tolerate this –

otherwise increase supplemental O_2 flow rate and/or improve overall ventilation. The recipient is unlikely to feel much better unless PaO_2 increases to at least 7.0–8.0 kPa.

HUMIDIFICATION

Humidification is not routinely required, but may be valuable in patients with tenacious secretions or rhinitis. A heat and moisture exchanger (e.g. Portex Thermovent) can be used, or for more intensive humidification, a heated water bath system (e.g. Fisher & Paykel) (see Fig. 10.1).

TOLERANCE OF NIPPV

Initially some patients may only be able to tolerate NIPPV for short periods. It helps to explore whether this is because ventilation is inadequate, the mask is uncomfortable or other medical problems have developed. However, where ventilatory efficiency has been optimized as far as possible, short periods of use are often better than nothing, so encourage the patient and gradually increase use – especially at night.

NIPPV FAILURE

This may occur in up to 20–40% of patients. If NIPPV cannot be made to work, it should be withdrawn while continuing with symptomatic measures, or the patient should be intubated if indicated.

PRACTICAL PROBLEMS

In one study [1] of the acute use of NIPPV the incidence of side-effects was:

mask discomfort 32%;
dry nose 20%;
air leaks 16%;
eye irritation 16%;
gastric distension 8%.

Not surprisingly, mask symptoms and nasal bridge sores increase when NIPPV is used intensively during a phase of acute illness and are less common during long-term nocturnal domiciliary use. By and large, side-effects do not cause NIPPV to be discontinued, but they do limit the efficiency of treatment.

NASAL BRIDGE SORES/PRESSURE NECROSIS (Fig. 5.1)

Pressure problems related to the mask are easier to prevent than cure. A carefully fitted mask, use of a polystyrene wedge or bubble mask (Rescare Ltd) to reduce pressure on the nasal bridge, and protective skin dressings such as Granuflex (ConvaTec Ltd) are useful preventive measures. If these fail, a switch to nasal plugs will usually allow the lesion to heal without stopping NIPPV. It is important to ensure that the patient is not ill-advisedly pulling the headgear straps too tight. For patients with recurrent pressure sores, an individually moulded mask or Silastic mask prothesis [2] may be needed. Patients receiving oral maintenance steroid therapy are at particular risk of developing skin ulceration [2].

RHINITIS, NASAL DRYNESS AND STREAMING

Minor nasal symptoms occur frequently in individuals new to NIPPV. Paradoxically, some experience nasal dryness and others nasal congestion and streaming. Short-term use of 0.5% ephedrine nose drops will reduce nasal congestion, and ipratropium nasal spray can relieve streaming. Long-term nasal steroid sprays have been used in patients with allergic rhinitis and persistent nasal symptoms. Others are helped by humidification. Nasal symptoms are exacerbated by mouth leaks and often lessen when the mouth leak is corrected.

MOUTH LEAKS (Fig. 5.2)

Mouth leaks during NIPPV occur frequently during wakefulness and sleep. Robert *et al.*

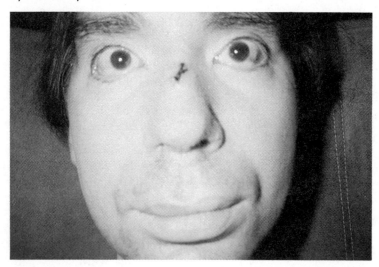

Fig. 5.1 Nasal bridge sore.

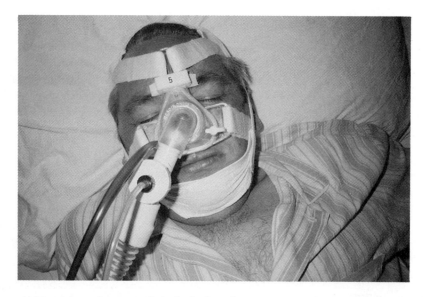

Fig. 5.2 Use of chin strap reduce mouth leak during sleep.

[3] carried out polysomnographic monitoring and showed that leaks from the mouth during sleep were responsible for increased arousals and poor ventilatory efficiency. Leaks around the top of the mask can lead to soreness of the eyes. The latter are best dealt with by improving the fit of the mask. Mouth leaks during sleep can be reduced by the patient using a chin strap, but often persist in mild form which may be overcome by increasing the level of ventilation. Mouth leaks in the initial period of NIPPV during an

acute exacerbation can cause serious under-ventilation. This is complicated by the fact that many patients in acute respiratory distress prefer to breathe through the mouth. This effectively bypasses a ventilator used with a nasal mask, as it will not be triggered in response to the patient's ventilatory efforts, and marked asynchrony ensues. For the patient this situation is not only inefficient but uncomfortable, as inspiratory efforts are unassociated with airflow and further machine-delivered breaths can cause hyper-inflation [4]. In such circumstances a full facemask is a better option.

As discussed in Chapter 3, pressure-preset equipment is better at compensating for leaks than volume-preset equipment.

GASTRIC DISTENSION

Abdominal bloating and gastric distension are often more sporadic than other side-effects. They tend to be more common in patients with high thoracic impedance and neuromuscular disease, and may respond to a change in position in bed. If this fails a temporary reduction in the flow rate or inspiratory pressure are helpful. Some patients swear by simple remedies such as charcoal biscuits, peppermint water, or alginate preparations.

AUTOPEEP

This is not a side-effect of NIPPV, but may pose particular problems in COPD patients. AutoPEEP or intrinsic end expiratory positive airway pressure (PEEPi) occurs in patients with severe airflow obstruction because of premature airway closure and air trapping and increases the work of breathing by adding an inspiratory threshold load (Chapter 2). In addition, it decreases effective trigger sensi-

tivity because PEEPi must be overcome before pressure change and flow occur and can be sensed at the nose. This may result in asynchrony between the patient's respiratory efforts and the machine breaths. This apparent asynchrony appears uncomfortable to the observer, but is usually well tolerated by the patient as inspiratory efforts do not result in airflow. As a consequence, subsequent gas delivery from the ventilator meets the patient's ventilatory requirements without causing breath stacking. However, the primary aim when starting NIPPV is to capture ventilation so that there is complete synchrony and minimal wasted effort. Measures directed at reducing bronchospasm, and possibly the use of low levels of EPAP may help, although the evidence to support this is more theoretical than real [5].

REFERENCES

1. Foglio, C., Vitacca, M., Quadri, A. *et al.* (1992) Acute exacerbations in severe COLD patients. Treatment using positive pressure ventilation by nasal mask. *Chest*, **101**, 1533–8.
2. Meecham Jones, D.J., Braid, G. and Wedzicha, J.A. (1994) Nasal masks for domiciliary positive pressure ventilation: patient usage and complications. *Thorax*, **49**, 811–12.
3. Robert, D., Langevin, B. and Leger, P. (1991) Mouth leaks during non-invasive nasal intermittent positive pressure ventilation (Abstract). Proceedings 3rd Conference on Pulmonary Rehabilitation and Home Ventilation, Denver, 1991, p. 99.
4. Branthwaite, M.A. (1991) Assisted ventilation 6. Non-invasive and domiciliary ventilation: positive pressure techniques. *Thorax*, **46**, 208–12.
5. Elliott, M.W. and Simonds, A.K. (1995) Nocturnal assisted ventilation using Bi-level positive airway pressure: the effect of expiratory positive airway pressure. *Eur. Respir. J.*, **8**, 436–40.

6

Non-invasive ventilation in the intensive care unit and operating theatre

JOHN C. GOLDSTONE

INTRODUCTION

Non-invasive positive pressure ventilation (NIPPV) has many attractive features which encourage its use within the intensive care unit (ICU). It has a potential role in the following situations.

- To avoid intubation in acute hypercapnic respiratory failure.
- In patients recovering from critical illness or sugery to circumvent the need for tracheostomy.
- To facilitate weaning.
- To improve preoperative cardiorespiratory function in patients with chronic ventilatory failure.

Additionally, in the field of anaesthesia, patients treated with long-term non-invasive ventilation may require surgery, which presents specific anaesthetic and ICU management problems.

Although negative pressure ventilation (nPV) has been employed in acute respiratory failure and to aid weaning, it is not available in many centres and far less flexible than NIPPV. NIPPV is more easily applied in the ICU and so discussion will be limited to this technique. Most published experience with NIPPV has been derived from the care of patients with chronic stable disease. Experience with NIPPV in the acute setting is less extensive.

NIPPV IN AVOIDANCE OF ENDOTRACHEAL INTUBATION

Endotracheal intubation has a number of physiological and practical disadvantages. General anaesthesia with neuromuscular blockade is required to facilitate intubation and this is associated with cardiovascular depression which is a dose-related response to the induction drugs and also related to the pre-intubation status of the patient, being enhanced by hypovolaemia. Further haemodynamic instability is produced by the pressor response to laryngoscopy and intubation. While several strategies have been adopted to attenuate this, the net effect on the myocardium is one of instability during the time

Non-Invasive Respiratory Support. Edited by Anita Simonds. Published by Chapman & Hall, London. ISBN 0412 56840 3.

mechanical ventilation is being instituted and it is not unusual for blood pressure to fall or rise in an uncontrolled manner.

In addition to these physiological effects, oral or nasal intubation requires the patient to be fed by nasogastric tube or parenterally, and limits communication and mobility. Mask ventilation avoids some of the adverse consequences of intubation, but there will always remain circumstances in which intubation is mandatory. Indications for endotracheal intubation are as follows.

- Patient deeply unconscious.
- Loss of bulbar reflexes.
- Risk of aspiration.
- Potential loss of upper airway (oedema, thermal injury etc.).

MASK TYPE

Nasal masks offer greater comfort and probably greater compliance in the chronic application of NIPPV; facemasks may be more effective in ICU patients. Continuous positive airway pressure (CPAP) therapy in the ICU is conventionally applied using a full facemask. Foglio and co-workers [1] showed no benefit of NIPPV over medical treatment in an early study, but their success increased in a subsequent study [2]. Brochard noted that this improvement may be attributable to the switch from nasal masks to facemasks [3].

NIPPV OR CPAP?

There have now been studies of the use of NIPPV in acute respiratory failure due to restrictive chest wall disease, neuromuscular disorders, COPD and cystic fibrosis (see Chapter 4). ICU staff also have extensive experience with CPAP in these situations. Data comparing CPAP and NIPPV are limited. Elliott *et al.* [4] showed that CPAP was less effective at improving oxygenation and reducing the work of breathing than NIPPV or pressure support in stable hypercapnic patients. However, a randomized trial [5] of CPAP, pressure support ventilation and volume-preset NIPPV in acute exacerbations of COPD has demonstrated improvement in PaO_2, with no difference between ventilatory modes, although control of $PaCO_2$ was variable. The immediate effects of CPAP in acute COPD have also been examined in an uncontrolled study by de Lucas *et al.* [6], who showed a significant increase in PaO_2, decrease in $PaCO_2$ and relief of dyspnoea. All patients received $5\,cmH_2O$ via a nasal mask and tolerated the CPAP well. However, both these latter studies were short term, lasting 1 and 4 hours respectively. Longer-term outcome is not given. Considering the information available, in practical terms a trial of CPAP may be helpful in the first instance, followed by NIPPV if CPAP proves unsatisfactory. In individuals with marked or rapidly escalating hypercapnia, NIPPV is probably the more logical option.

An important consequence of using non-invasive respiratory support is that ITU beds may be saved as non-intubated patients can be managed on a high dependency unit or general ward [7]. Bott *et al.* [7] found that NIPPV was well accepted by nursing staff and that no additional staff were required. Another substantial benefit of NIPPV is that the patients do not receive ventilation continuously, and many are able to mobilize between treatments. Vitacca and others found that NIPPV was required for 16 hours in the first day and this could be decreased to 10 hours on the second day [2].

Intubation may become necessary in acute respiratory failure, despite NIPPV. An intubation rate of up to 20% may occur, although the need for intubation arose after 80 hours of NIPPV in one study [2]. Endotracheal intubation results in a more prolonged ICU admission, possibly because of the increased severity of disease [8].

NIPPV IN AVOIDANCE OF TRACHEOSTOMY

Endotracheal intubation facilitates mechanical ventilation of the lungs, and with careful management it is possible to maintain this airway over a number of weeks. For many patients the presence of the endotracheal tube (ET) requires sedation. When sedation is provided solely because of the presence of an endotracheal tube there is a clear advantage to alternative methods of airway control. Decisions concerning the airway in these patients generally depend on how quickly spontaneous respiration recovers. Extubation and institution of non-invasive support avoids tracheostomy and enables the patient to recover airway control. Potential benefits of this approach included aided mucociliary clearance, effective spontaneous coughing and restoring the nasal route for ventilation (humidification and a decrease in resistive work). Early extubation removes the ET tube as a portal of entry for pathogens.

DISADVANTAGES OF TRACHEOSTOMY

- Surgical procedure which requires sedation/general anaesthesia.
- Bleeding [9].
- Loss of airway control.
- Infection at the tracheostomy site.
- Later complications, e.g. stenosis.

The work performed through artificial airways is complex and is related to the presence of turbulent rather than laminar flow, the diameter and length of the airway itself and the obstruction created by deformation or debris on the wall of the tube [10]. Because the determinants of the work of breathing through an artificial airway are related to these other factors in addition to the diameter and length of the tube, it is not always the case that tracheostomy tubes offer a decrease in the work performed during breathing [11]. In individual patients the tracheostomy itself may distort the airway, and the more rigid types may impact on the posterior wall of the trachea, further obstructing the airway. Occasionally removal of the tracheostomy tube may facilitate spontaneous breathing [12].

Percutaneous tracheostomy is a relatively new method which may reduce immediate morbidity [13,14]. During dilatation of the trachea there is a technical advantage to placing smaller tracheostomy tubes, reducing the force required and final size of dilator. Tube size as a determinant of resistive work across the airway becomes increasingly important as inspiratory flow increases. It is important that the patient should not be expected to breathe spontaneously through a small tube.

NIPPV IN WEANING FROM MECHANICAL VENTILATION

Failure to wean from mechanical ventilation occurs in a minority of patients who then require days or weeks of further treatment, often at a time in their illness when other organ systems are recovering and the general level of care is declining [15]. This small group of 'difficult to wean' patients require considerable attention. Spontaneous breathing requires an adequate central nervous system output relative to the strength of the respiratory muscles in the face of the applied load during each breath. In those who are difficult to wean, optimization of these three components (CNS drive, respiratory muscle strength and the applied load) is often the key to further progress. This group of patients can be considered as being in a controlled form of respiratory failure where the function of the respiratory muscle 'pump' is offloaded by the ventilator.

CENTRAL NERVOUS SYSTEM DRIVE

This can be profoundly affected by sedative and general anaesthetic drugs. Whereas 'normal' patients can compensate for sedative drugs, those patients in respiratory failure suffer a sharp decline in ventilatory function, as they are more dependent on respiratory drive. When measured in weaning patients, respiratory drive is usually increased, especially in individuals who fail and are making even greater efforts to breathe [16].

THE LOAD APPLIED TO THE SYSTEM

Load is increased by endotracheal intubation [17]. If the respiratory rate and minute ventilation is high, which is common in patients who fail to wean, the load imposed by the ET tube can approach that which would exhaust a normal subject [18]. Further changes occur in ET tube resistance if there are kinks or deposits on the surface of the tube, decreasing the functional diameter.

THE PATIENT : VENTILATOR INTERFACE

Although many ventilator modes require the patient to initiate a breath ('triggering'), this does not mean that the inspiratory muscles only contract during this time [19]. Rather, contraction occurs during the majority of the inspiratory cycle and the potential therefore exists that the respiratory muscles get less benefit than during controlled mechanical ventilation. This is related in part to the ability of the ventilator to sense the beginning of ventilation. Many ventilators begin the inspiratory cycle when the pressure within the ventilator achieves a pre-set level. The transmission of intrathoracic pressure to the ventilator will be impaired by the presence of any resistance between the respiratory muscles and the ventilator, and this would include resistance within the endotracheal tube as well as intrapulmonary resistances. The characteristics of the ventilator are important when optimizing treatment for a patient who is difficult to wean. It is important that the ventilator responds rapidly to a minimal change in pressure. Triggering the ventilator to operate when flow occurs within the tubing may be advantageous.

THE STRENGTH OF THE RESPIRATORY MUSCLES

Patients recovering after critical illness are often weak, and when the respiratory muscles are tested a 70% reduction in strength is often noted [20]. In order to achieve gas flow at the mouth, intrathoracic pressure must be predominantly negative. In respiratory disease a resting positive alveolar pressure exists (autoPEEP effect) and this may be worsened by apparatus which further impedes expiratory gas flow. The respiratory muscles therefore have to generate a negative pressure which exceeds autoPEEP before gas flows and this 'threshold load' can exceed 10–15 cmH$_2$O. Any reduction in load achieved by decreasing autoPEEP will be beneficial. In the setting of a weak patient threshold load is particularly relevant, as some patients will be expected to generate some 50% of their maximum strength merely to achieve gas flow at the mouth. Experimental evidence from normal subjects [21] and from weaning patients [22] suggests that when the ratio of pressure required per breath to maximum pressure exceeds 40%, spontaneous breathing cannot be sustained. In this group of patients improvement would be expected from a decrease in threshold load. This can be achieved by removing added resistances such as the ET tube.

INTRODUCING NIPPV TO THE INTUBATED PATIENT

Patients often become accustomed to a pattern of ventilation produced by a particular ventilator and this is especially noticeable when the mode of ventilation is changed (i.e. from pressure- to volume-limited). Several

53

of the common dedicated NIPPV devices deliver pre-set volumes whereas spontaneously breathing patients are often attached to pressure-controlled modes of ventilation. For this reason, patients should be allowed to try the NIPPV ventilator before decannulation for a period of acclimatization before face-mask ventilation is delivered. This enables the ventilator to be individually adjusted, remembering that higher pre-set tidal volumes will be required after extubation because of gas leakage from around the mask and an increase in upper airway deadspace.

It is our practice to provide NIPPV initially with a facemask, and a suggested sequence of events is given below. Many patients require reassurance at this stage and it is not infrequent that NIPPV has to be applied in stages. It is essential that the medical staff have a clear understanding of the device and its application. This can be extended to include a team of doctors, nurses any physiotherapists to enable NIPPV to be applied successfully throughout the day and night. Although the dedicated devices are generally less complex than ICU ventilators, it is not the case that the application of this treatment is simple.

Suggested sequence to initiate NIPPV in a previously ventilated patient

- It is sensible to wait until the tracheostomy tract is mature (i.e. >3 days following stoma creation) to reduce the risk of subcutaneous emphysema.
- Begin with initiating NIPPV via the tracheostomy/endotracheal tube to ensure that satisfactory arterial blood gas control can be achieved using the ventilator which is to be used with the mask system.
- If the patient has a tracheostomy, facemask ventilation is given with the cuff deflated and the tracheostomy closed prior to decannulation.
- Decannulation can be achieved rapidly in most patients after 12–24 hours' successful mask ventilation.

- The stoma can be sealed with occlusive tape until healing occurs.
- NIPPV is particularly acceptable if the patient can manage off the ITU ventilator for short periods, e.g. 5 minutes. It should not be initiated in an individual who is entirely ventilator-dependent.

OUTCOME OF NIPPV TO FACILITATE WEANING

Udwadia and colleagues studied 22 patients with restrictive or obstructive disorders who were referred to a specialist chronic ventilation unit for weaning from mechanical ventilation [23]. NIPPV was well tolerated in 20 patients and 18 of these were extubated or decannulated quickly. The period of time between initiation of NIPPV and discharge home was brief (median 11 days) compared to the previous duration of conventional IPPV (median 31 days) (Fig. 6.1). All patients were transferred to a general ward within 24 hours of starting NIPPV. Ten patients remained nasally ventilated at night when discharged home. Of the eight patients who received no support, four were prescribed protriptyline to control nocturnal hypoventilation. In another series NIPPV was used effectively in 13/14 patients with weaning problems due to COPD or chest wall disease [24]. Most COPD patients did not require long-term ventilatory support. Although these studies were not controlled they demonstrate that difficult-to-wean patients can be successfully extubated or decannulated using NIPPV. Patients with chest wall disorders appear more likely to need long-term respiratory support after weaning than those with COPD.

NIPPV TO IMPROVE PREOPERATIVE CARDIORESPIRATORY FUNCTION [25]

Patients with impaired preoperative function withstand surgery poorly. When time allows, a course of NIPPV may potentially reduce these risks. Familiarization with the tech-

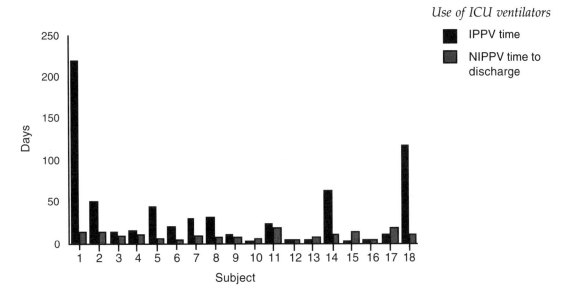

Fig. 6.1 Outcome of NIPPV in weaning from mechanical ventilation. (Reproduced with permission from Udwadia *et al.* [23]).

nique is also helpful as patients are likely to benefit from an additional period of non-invasive ventilation in the postoperative period. There are no studies of the physiological effects and cost-effectiveness of NIPPV applied in this way.

NON-INVASIVE VENTILATION WITH ICU VENTILATORS

Non-invasive ventilation has frequently been delivered by conventional ventilators [26–28], although specialized NIPPV devices are now available, as described in Chapter 3. The use of this technique to provide nocturnal and domiciliary ventilation necessitates ventilators which are robust and simple to use for home use. In the UK access to dedicated non-invasive devices is not widespread in ICUs. Although some centres have demonstrated that non-invasive techniques do not require intensive or even high dependency care, it may be the case that staffing levels and skill-mixes of general wards do not enable this technique to be contemplated. As a con-

sequence, it is likely that initial experience of non-invasive ventilation within non-specialist hospitals will occur within ITU/high dependency areas. This raises the question: can NIPPV be provided by existing conventional mechanical ventilators?

We have recently measured the characteristics of two ITU ventilators and compared this to a commonly available non-invasive device designed for home ventilation. We measured the timing of inspiration from the beginning of negative pressure generation in the chest with an oesophageal ballon catheter to the point when inspiratory flow began at the airway. We also quantified the work performed to initiate each breath by measuring the area of the oesophageal waveform during inspiration, the pressure time index.

Figure 6.2 demonstrates a typical tracing in a normal subject ventilated through a face-mask with the three ventilators. The time delay was greatest in the Servo 900C whereas there was little difference between the Puritan Bennett 7200 and the NIPPV ventilator, the BromptonPAC. When the effort required to initiate each breath is compared there is a

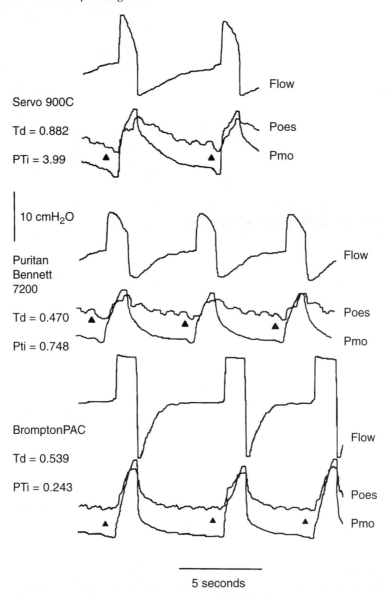

5 seconds

Fig. 6.2 Two typical ITU ventilators (Siemens Servo 900C and Puritan Bennett 7200) were compared to a specially designed NIPPV device (BromptonPAC) in normal subjects ventilated through a facemask. A representative tracing from a single subject shows flow, oesophageal (Poes) and mouth (Pmo) pressures during ventilation with inspiratory pressure support of $10\,cmH_2O$ (Servo 900C and Puritan Bennett) and volume preset ventilation adjusted to the same tidal volume. The arrowheads denote the onset of inspiration. Average time delay (Td) between the onset of inspiration and inspiratory flow at the mouth is given for each ventilator. The average pressure time index of the oesophageal waveform (PTi), an indicator of the work performed to initiate the breath, is also given.

tenfold difference between the Servo 900C and the BromptonPAC.

The mode of ventilation is also important when setting an ICU ventilator to be used non-invasively. In spontaneously breathing intubated patients, inspiratory pressure support (IPS) has become popular. Especially when using the nasal route to deliver support, pressure-support ventilation delivers high gas flows when the airway is partially open and this may be uncomfortable when the gas expands the patient's nasal airways. An additional problem with IPS is that the mechanical breath is often terminated by the reduction of flow rate at the end of inspiration (often when this reduces to 25% of initial flow rate). If the leak of gas continues, inspiration is prolonged unless the subject performs a forced expiration through the nose, actively terminating the breath. For these reasons, IPS is easier to administer through a facemask.

Figure 6.3 demonstrates our results when a different mode of ventilation is selected. In this example, volume pre-set breaths are shown. Although the Servo 900C is still worse in terms of breath initiation, it is substantially better in this mode when compared to pressure support. It would appear that improvements can be obtained in different ventilator modes in individual cases.

ANAESTHESIA FOR PATIENTS DEPENDENT ON NON-INVASIVE VENTILATION

PREOPERATIVE ASSESSMENT

It is fundamentally important to characterize the underlying disease. The indications for NIPPV vary and while few patients are ventilated for obstructive lung disease in the UK there is considerable experience overseas. NIPPV is provided for a range of illnesses, including neuromuscular disease, restrictive disease of the chest wall and obstructive lung disease. Children are less commonly treated with NIPPV but may require incidental surgery for orthopaedic or airway problems.

Cardiorespiratory function should be fully assessed, the requirements for added oxygen noted and the presence of pulmonary hypertension sought. Arterial blood gas tensions should be optimized as far as possible. Many patients require NIPPV at night and can adequately ventilate during the day. The ability to breathe unsupported makes continuous postoperative ventilation less likely provided important changes in respiratory mechanics, lung volume, intravascular volume and CNS drive are avoided. The patient's home ventilator should *always* be available in the postoperative period, and recovery room and anaesthetic staff familiarized with its operation.

ANAESTHETIC MANAGEMENT

Sedation prior to anaesthesia is generally contraindicated and should only be contemplated under monitored conditions. The addition of supplemental oxygen may also reduce ventilatory drive. Supine posture may worsen gas exchange and promote orthopnoea in those patients who are weak.

Difficulty in intubation occasionally occurs in patients with chest wall deformity and these individuals should be assessed in the standard manner when problems are anticipated.

The choice between spontaneous breathing and mechanical ventilation is only relevant in the shortest of procedures and in all other cases controlled breathing is preferable. General anaesthesia will reduce central nervous system drive and ventilation is further reduced by a disadvantageous posture.

The conduct of mechanical ventilation is important in that hyperinflation worsens intrinsic or autoPEEP and further hyperinflation shortens the respiratory muscles, leading to a decrease in their ability to shorten and generate tension. While restrictive lung dis-

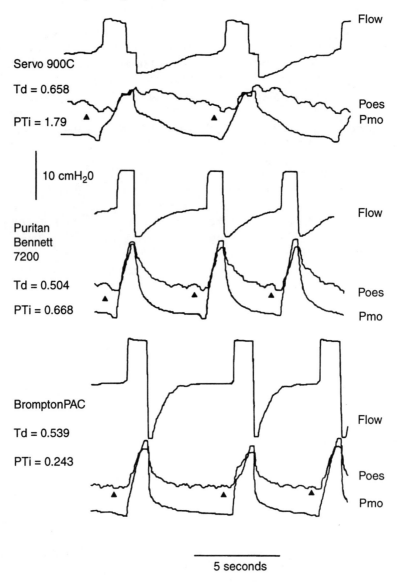

Fig. 6.3 Two typical ITU ventilators – Siemens Servo 900C (SIMV) and Puritan Bennett 7200 (assist-control) – were compared to a specifically designed NIPPV device (BromptonPAC) in normal subjects ventilated through a facemask. Average values are shown for the time delay in initiating ventilation (Td) and the effort required to initiate ventilation (PTi). The arrowheads denote the onset of inspiration.

ease often represents an increase in work above the tidal volume range, the pressure required to inflate the lungs is surprisingly normal.

There is little evidence that the anaesthetic technique itself is of importance and differences between techniques and drugs are likely to be small.

Table 6.1 Monitoring during anaesthesia

Variable	End-point
$PaCO_2$	Ventilation to preoperative $PaCO_2$
	End-tidal CO_2 may be misleading in severe obstructive lung disease
AutoPeep	Ensure no rise. Avoid hyperinflation during anaesthesia
Central venous pressure (CVP)	Right heart function should be monitored with CVP line
Pulmonary artery (PA) pressure	PA catheterization if pulmonary hypertension likely and severe
Twitch height and response to tetanic stimulation	Recovery of full motor power

Monitoring should be adapted to individual circumstances. In addition to standard monitoring of arterial oxygen saturation and vital signs, measurement of the variables listed in Table 6.1 should be considered.

POSTOPERATIVE CARE

A return to the preoperative level of ventilatory support, using the patient's domiciliary equipment, should be the target but it is important to be realistic about the chances of success. Intra-abdominal and intrathoracic procedures which generally compromise ventilation will be even more deleterious than in normal subjects and it may not be possible to manage postoperative pain effectively with epidural anaesthesia in the face of skeletal deformity. Patients should be extubated and receive non-invasive support as soon as acute problems resolve. Recovery and postoperative care should be carefully monitored.

REFERENCES

1. Foglio, C., Vitacca, M., Quadri, A. *et al.* (1992) Acute exacerbations in severe COLD patients. Treatment using positive pressure ventilation by nasal mask. *Chest*, **101**, 1533–8.
2. Vitacca, M., Ribini, F., Foglio, K. *et al.* (1993) Non-invasive modalities of positive pressure ventilation improve the outcome of acute exacerbations in COLD patients. *Intens. Care Med.*, **19**, 450–5.
3. Brochard, L. (1993) Non-invasive ventilation: practice issues (Editorial comment). *Intens. Care. Med.*, **19**, 431–2.
4. Elliott, M.W., Aquilina, R., Green, M. *et al.* (1994) A comparison of different modes of noninvasive respiratory support: effects on ventilation and inspiratory muscle effort. *Anaesthesia*, **49**, 279–83.
5. Meecham Jones, D.J., Paul, E.A., Graham-Clarke, C. and Wedzicha, J.A. (1994) Nasal ventilation in acute exacerbations of chronic obstructive pulmonary disease: effect of ventilator mode on arterial blood gas tensions. *Thorax*, **49**, 1222–4.
6. de Lucas, P., Tarancon, C., Puente, L. *et al.* (1993) Nasal continuous positive airway pressure in patients with COPD in acute respiratory failure. A study of the immediate effects. *Chest*, **104**, 1694–7.
7. Bott, J., Carroll, M.P., Conway, J.H. *et al.* (1993) Randomised controlled trial of nasal ventilation in acute ventilatory failure due to chronic obstructive airways disease. *Lancet*, **341**, 1555–7.
8. Fernandez, R., Blanch, L., Valles, J. *et al.* (1993) Pressure support ventilation via face mask in acute respiratory failure in hypercapnic COPD patients. *Intens. Care Med.*, **19**, 456–61.
9. Stanffer, J.L. and Silvestri, R.C. (1982) Complications of endotracheal intubation, tracheostomy and artificial airways. *Respiratory Care*, **27**, 417–34.
10. Habib, M.P. (1989) Physiological implications of artificial airways. *Chest*, **96**, 181–4.
11. Plost, J. and Cabell, J.C. (1984) The non-elastic work of breathing through endotracheal tubes of various sizes. *Am. Rev. Respir. Dis.*, **129**, A106.

12. Criner, G., Make, B. and Celli, B. (1987) Respiratory muscle dysfunction secondary to chronic tracheostomy tube placement. *Chest*, **91**, 139–41.

13. Ciaglia, P., Firshing, R. and Syniec, C. (1985) Elective percutaneous dilatational tracheostomy. A new simple bedside procedure; preliminary report. *Chest*, **87**, 715–19.

14. Hazard, P., Jones, C. and Benitone, J. (1991) Comparative clinical trial of standard operative tracheostomy with percutaneous tracheostomy. *Crit. Care Med.*, **19**, 1018–24.

15. Morganroth, M.L., Morganroth, J.L. and Nett, L.M. (1984) Criteria for weaning from prolonged mechanical ventilation. *Arch. Intern. Med.*, **144**, 1012–16.

16. Herrera, M., Blasco, J., Venegas, J. *et al.* (1985) Mouth occlusion pressure (PO.1) in acute respiratory failure. *Intens. Care Med.*, **11**, 134–9.

17. Wright, P.E., Marini, J.J. and Bernard, G.R. (1989) *In vitro* versus *in vivo* comparison of endotracheal tube airflow resistance. *Am. Rev. Respir. Dis.*, **140**, 10–16.

18. Shapiro, M., Wilson, R.K., Casar, G. *et al.* (1986) Work of breathing through different sized endotracheal tubes. *Crit. Care Med.*, **14**, 1028–31.

19. Marini, J., Capps, J.S. and Culver, B.H.J. (1985) The inspiratory work of breathing during assisted mechanical ventilation. *Chest*, **87**, 612–18.

20. Kacmarek, R.M., Cycyk-Chapman, M.C., Young-Palazzo, P.J. and Romagnoli, D.M. (1989) Determination of maximum inspiratory pressure: a clinical study and literature review. *Respiratory Care*, **34**, 868–78.

21. Roussos, C.S. and Macklem, P.T. (1977) Diaphragmatic fatigue in man. *J. Appl. Physiol.*, **43**, 189–97.

22. Goldstone, J.C., Green, M. and Moxham, J. (1994) Maximum relaxation rate of the diaphragm during weaning from mechanical ventilation. *Thorax*, **49**, 54–60.

23. Udwadia, Z.F., Santis, G.F., Steven, M.H. and Simonds, A.K. (1992) Nasal ventilation to facilitate weaning in patients with chronic respiratory insufficiency. *Thorax*, **47**(9): 715–18.

24. Restrick, L.J., Scott, A.D., Ward, A.D. *et al.* (1993) Nasal intermittent positive-pressure ventilation in weaning intubated patients with chronic respiratory disease from assisted intermittent positive-pressure ventilation. *Respir. Med.*, **87**, 199–204.

25. Simonds, A.K. (1994) Non-invasive respiratory support: intensive care applications. *Br. J. Intens. Care*, **4**, 235–41.

26. Marino, W. (1991) Intermittent volume cycled mechanical ventilation via nasal mask in patients with respiratory failure due to COPD. *Chest*, **99**, 681–4.

27. Meduri, G.U., Abou-Shala, N., Fox, R.C. *et al.* (1991) Non-invasive facemask mechanical ventilation in patients with acute hypercapnic respiratory failure. *Chest*, **100**, 445–54.

28. Bach, J.R., Alba, A., Mosher, R. and Delaubier, A. (1987) Intermittent positive pressure ventilation via nasal access in the management of respiratory insufficiency. *Chest*, **92**(1): 168–70.

7

Selection of patients for home ventilation

ANITA K. SIMONDS

INTRODUCTION

Assisted ventilation may be required long term in the home or for a short period during an exacerbation of chronic respiratory failure. In general, ventilatory dependency can be classified into four categories.

Grade 1   Assisted ventilation required after an acute illness or operation.
Grade 2   Assisted ventilation required regularly during sleep.
Grade 3   Assisted ventilation required during sleep and some part of the day.
Grade 4   Assisted ventilation required continuously.

The majority of patients using non-invasive ventilation at home in the United Kingdom fall into categories 2 and 3. A small proportion require ventilation continuously and almost all these grade 4 patients are treated with tracheostomy–IPPV, although a handful continue treatment with NIPPV or in the iron lung. The number of patients in category 1 who receive treatment for an acute hypercapnic exacerbation is unknown, but is certainly growing as more units begin to employ non-invasive ventilatory techniques.

Benefit from home ventilation has been demonstrated in the following conditions.

1. Treatment of hypercapnic respiratory failure due to:
   - Chest wall disease
     Scoliosis
     Thoracoplasty
     Fibrothorax
   - Respiratory muscle disorders
     Old poliomyelitis
     Myopathies
     Muscular dystrophies
   - Neurological disorders
     Primary alveolar hypoventilation
     Central sleep apnoea
     Brain stem lesions
     Cervical spinal cord injury
     Phrenic nerve lesions
     Polyneuropathy
2. Possible indications (see text)
   - COPD
   - Bronchiectasis
   - Rapidly progressive neuromuscular disease

Information on the outcome of home ventilation in these groups is given in Chapter 8 and 9. Here the indications for starting elective

Non-Invasive Respiratory Support. Edited by Anita Simonds. Published by Chapman & Hall, London. ISBN 0412 56840 3.

domiciliary non-invasive ventilation are discussed.

ELECTIVE INDICATIONS

Starting home ventilation is a major under-taking for the patient and his/her family which has major social and financial im-plications. The appropriate timing of this intervention is therefore crucial. The elective introduction of any treatment presupposes that high-risk patients can be identified, and the natural history of the underlying re-spiratory disorder is known. This entails appropriate monitoring of the patient to detect trends in pulmonary function. Clearly, it is essential that all standard therapeutic options have been fully explored before em-barking on respiratory support. Each of these aspects will be considered in turn.

IDENTIFICATION OF PATIENTS AT HIGH RISK OF VENTILATORY FAILURE

Several longitudinal studies [1–3] have con-firmed the excess morbidity and premature mortality associated with severe unfused idiopathic scoliosis. Cor pulmonale was the primary cause of death in 30% of 102 patients with untreated idiopathic scoliosis followed for 50 years [2] (Chapter 2).

Branthwaite [3] has shown that patients with unfused idiopathic scoliosis and a vital capacity of less than 50% predicted at pre-sentation may develop a disproportionate loss of lung volume with age. By contrast, patients with a vital capacity of more than 50% predicted were unlikely to develop respiratory problems (Fig. 7.1). The age of onset of scoliosis is important, with those acquiring the curvature at less than 5 years of age being at most risk of cardiorespiratory decompensation. Here, the early onset of the deformity may restrict alveolar duplication and the maturation of pulmonary vasculature. In addition, congenital scoliosis may be as-

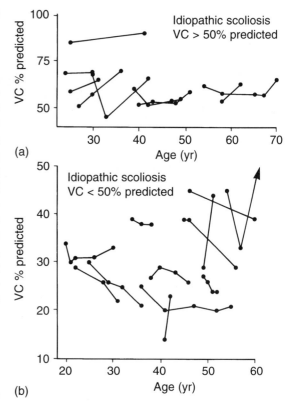

(a)

(b)

Fig. 7.1 Longitudinal trends in patients with early onset unfused idiopathic scoliosis with vital capa-city at presentation (a) less than 50% predicted, (b) greater than 50% predicted. The three subjects who show an increase in VC received NIPPV. (Reproduced from Branthwaite [3]).

sociated with other disorders, including congenital heart defects. In a separate study of mortality, over 90% of individuals who experienced cardiorespiratory failure which could be attributed to the scoliosis, developed their thoracic deformity at less than 5 years of age. A high thoracic curve seems to have a more adverse prognosis than a low thoracic defect, probably because it places the re-spiratory muscles and rib cage at a greater mechanical disadvantage.

In confirmation of some of these findings, Pehrsson [4] has reported results from a 20-year follow-up of lung function in adult idiopathic scoliosis. Respiratory failure occurred in 25% of patients (6 out of 24). All those who developed respiratory failure had a vital capacity of less than 45% predicted and a thoracic spinal curvature which exceeded 110°. Wheeze was more common in those who decompensated, although most patients did not smoke. The presence of additional respiratory pathology, such as asthma, may be sufficient to precipitate respiratory failure in those with borderline function. The peak incidence of respiratory failure in the UK series [3] was during the fifth decade, although in this study and the Swedish series the age at decompensation ranged widely from 30 to 70 years.

Considering the evolution of respiratory failure in other conditions, an analysis of 180 patients requiring NIPPV at the Royal Brompton Hospital [5] has shown that the mean age (range) at which NIPPV was initiated for patients with previous poliomyelitis was 51.2 (25–76) years, for sequelae of pulmonary tuberculosis, 61.8 (45–75) years, for COPD, 58.2 (42–72) years, and for bronchiectasis, 39.8 (19–61) years. In this cohort the mean age of patients with early onset idiopathic scoliosis when starting NIPPV was 49.1 years (range 17–74 years). Pulmonary function tests demonstrated a mean (s.d.) vital capacity of 0.82 (0.37) litres in the early onset scoliosis patients, 1.1 (0.4) litres in poliomyelitis patients, and 1.2 (0.6) litres in those with previous tuberculosis. In the group with obstructive lung disease, mean (s.d.) FEV_1 was 0.58 (0.3) litres in COPD patients and 0.48 (0.16) litres in those with bronchiectasis.

Respiration during sleep has been compared in patients with scolioses of varying aetiology [6]. Nocturnal arterial oxygen saturation was lowest in patients with a paralytic scoliosis associated with a severe reduction in vital capacity, and in older patients with non-paralytic scoliosis. The degree of scoliosis did not correlate well with the extent of nocturnal desaturation. In patients with neuromuscular disease, minimum arterial oxygen saturation during sleep was correlated with vital capacity, and the percentage fall in vital capacity on changing from the erect to supine position. There was a relationship between daytime arterial blood gas tensions and nocturnal desaturation, but the wide scatter in results makes it difficult to predict the degree of nocturnal desaturation on the basis of diurnal values alone. In this study, maximum inspiratory mouth pressures were not correlated with nocturnal saturation.

Braun *et al.* [7] have demonstrated that in patients with neuromuscular disorders a vital capacity of less than 55% predicted and mouth pressures of less than 30% strongly predict the development of daytime hypercapnia.

Regarding high-risk COPD patients, there is a clear relationship between the degree of airflow obstruction and the risk of cardiorespiratory failure. However, the predictive value of FEV_1 for nocturnal desaturation is not high, and the best predictor of oxygenation during sleep is awake arterial oxygen saturation. The presence of obstructive sleep apnoea in addition can produce profound nocturnal desaturation.

MONITORING

Having identified high-risk patients, the purpose of follow-up is to detect a progressive fall in lung volumes and the development of nocturnal hypoventilation, before progression to frank diurnal respiratory failure and cor pulmonale occurs. Early diagnosis and intervention is important as evidence suggests that the outcome of nocturnal ventilation is less good in those with longstanding cor pulmonale and pulmonary hypertension [5]. As a routine, standard treatment measures can be optimized and advice given regarding general health, including ideal body weight. Weight gain with age is an important hazard in patients with limited respiratory reserve. Hormone replacement therapy is probably advisable in post-menopausal female scoliotic patients to prevent the development of osteoporosis and progression of the curvature. In most patients the presence of morning headache, fatigue and poor sleep quality correlates well with the degree of nocturnal hypoventilation. A headache on waking may be wrongly ascribed to musculoskeletal pain resulting from a cervical scoliosis. A hypercapnic, scoliotic female was recently referred to the author's unit who had undergone temporal artery biopsy and CT scan of the brain before arterial blood gas measurement was considered.

Some patients may present with nocturnal confusion and overt psychiatric features, although this is uncommon [8]. For example, a patient referred with severe respiratory muscle weakness due to motor neurone disease presented with temper tantrums and confusion on waking associated with profound hypercapnic respiratory failure.

Following questioning about symptoms, routine assessment should include pulmonary function tests, measurement of arterial blood gas tensions and the monitoring of respiration during sleep. A progressive fall in lung volumes (notably vital capacity and total lung capacity) is usually seen in restrictive disorders. In individuals with mild to moderate nocturnal hypoventilation prior to the development of overt diurnal respiratory failure a raised base excess is frequently observed and should prompt overnight investigation. Nocturnal monitoring in this situation should include oximetry and either transcutanous or end-tidal CO_2. End-tidal CO_2 measurements are relatively reliable in patients with restrictive disorders, but do not accurately represent alveolar P_{CO_2} in subjects with severe airflow obstruction. Transcutaneous CO_2 measurement has been found to follow changes in arterial P_{CO_2} reliably [9], although some workers dispute this [10]. The response time

of the electrode is inevitably slower than oximetry so that a maximum reading represents the peak level achieved during an episode of hypoventilation rather than an accurate representation of CO_2 fluctuations during individual hypopnoeas. Additional monitoring of chest wall movement and oronasal airflow is helpful to characterize apnoea and hypopnoeas, especially in conditions such as Duchenne muscular dystrophy and motor neurone disease where bulbar weakness predisposes the individual to upper airway obstruction. Full polysomnography is not essential, but it is important that at least some probable REM sleep is observed, as early nocturnal hypoventilation will always be manifest in this sleep stage [11] (Chapter 2). Clinical practice has shown that diurnal respiratory failure in the presence of preserved inspiratory muscle strength ($>70\,cmH_2O$) is highly suggestive of a significant component of upper airway obstruction during sleep [11].

Global respiratory muscle strength is best measured using a mouth pressure meter (e.g. Precision Medical Ltd, Pickering, Yorkshire) (Fig. 7.2). Using this device, expiratory muscle strength (PE_{max}) is measured at the mouth as the patient makes a maximum expiratory effort against a closed airway from total lung capacity. Likewise, inspiratory muscle strength (PI_{max}) can be gauged from the pressure obtained at the mouth during a maximum inspiratory effort from residual volume or functional residual capacity. The meter includes a small leak to prevent erroneously high pressures being generated by the buccal muscles. Accurate measurement depends on careful explanation of the technique and full patient cooperation.

Reference normal ranges depend on the sort of mouthpiece used, but a PI_{max} above $80\,cmH_2O$ excludes significant weakness of the inspiratory muscles [12].

A more detailed assessment of diaphragm muscle function can be obtained by passage

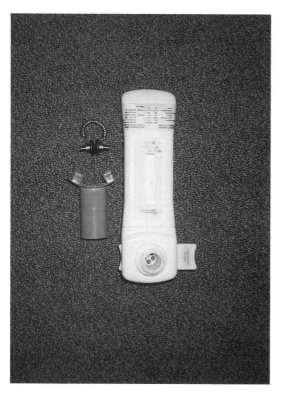

Fig. 7.2 Mouth pressure meter for measuring PI_{max} and PE_{max} (Precision Medical Ltd).

of an oesophageal ballon to measure transdiaphragmatic pressure. In the presence of a low transdiaphragmatic pressure, phrenic nerve stimulation in the neck will clarify the functional integrity of the phrenic nerves. Both measurement of mouth pressure and transdiaphragmatic pressure during maximal voluntary effort is dependent on patient co-operation. Cervical root excitation using a magnetic stimulator over C3–5 and transcutaneous phrenic nerve stimulation in the supraclavicular fossa both avoid a volitional element and may be useful to confirm true weakness, when poor effort is suspected.

During follow-up the motivation of the patient and social and psychological factors can be assessed and the individual and family prepared for the introduction of home ventilation. Patients often find it helpful to meet other individuals who are already using home ventilation.

TREATMENT OPTIONS FOR VENTILATORY INSUFFICIENCY

There are a number of treatments which are worth exploring in patients with stable hypercapnia and mild to moderate nocturnal hypoventilation. These may allow the use of home ventilation to be avoided or delayed for up to several years.

Drug therapy

The tricyclic drug protriptyline can control moderate nocturnal hypoventilation [13,14] and is usually more successful in restrictive disorders than COPD. It appears to work by reducing REM sleep-related hypoventilation, although an independent effect on upper airway tone may play a part [15]. Low doses (5–10 mg at night) are sufficient. Higher doses (as used to treat depression) are associated with significant anticholinergic side-effects, including dry mouth, constipation, urinary hesitancy and impotence. Protriptyline should be given with caution in individuals with a history of prostatism, and all users should be warned of the risk of photosensitivity. It is not possible to predict which individuals will respond to protriptyline. In some patients improvement in nocturnal and diurnal arterial blood gas tension is maintained over years [16], while in others the effect is transient [17], or side-effects preclude long-term use [14].

Almitrine has been shown to produce a sustained increase in nocturnal and diurnal oxygenation in COPD patients. The precise mechanism of action is unclear, but almitrine has been shown to have a stimulant effect on carotid and aortic body chemoreceptors [18] and improves ventilation–perfusion matching by a direct effect on the pulmonary vascular bed [19]. In many countries, however, the drug is not freely prescribable.

Medroxyprogesterone stimulates hypercapnic ventilatory drive during wakefulness and sleep, and can produce a small fall in $PaCO_2$ in some patients with chronic respiratory failure [20]. However, side-effects including fluid retention and impotence in males limit its application.

Acetazolamide increases urinary bicarbonate ion excretion and shifts the ventilatory response to hypercapnia to the left. Occasional short-term benefit has been seen in patients with hypercapnic COPD [21], although care should be taken to avoid worsening the level of acidosis. Acetazolamide may have a minor role in central sleep apnoea [22], but as with other respiratory stimulants, side-effects are troublesome.

Long-term oxygen therapy

According to the guidelines for England and Wales for the prescription of long-term oxygen therapy, LTOT is the treatment of choice in COPD patients who fulfil the following criteria.

1. Patients with chronic obstructive pulmonary disease
   with an FEV_1 less than 1.5 litres
        FVC   less than 2.0 litres
        PaO_2 less than 7.3 kPa
   with hypercapnia and a history of oedema
2. COPD patients as in (1) but without hypercapnia or oedema.
3. As palliation of pre-terminal respiratory failure of any aetiology with PaO_2 less than 7.3 kPa.

   Measurements of PaO_2 should be made when patients are stable. PaO_2 should be less than 7.3 kPa on two occasions at least 3 weeks apart.

Until the results of trials comparing nocturnal nasal ventilation and LTOT in COPD are available, LTOT should be first line tretament and nasal ventilation considered only in hypercapnic COPD patients who tolerate oxygen therapy poorly (see Chapter 9). LTOT is usually inadvisable in severe restrictive disorders because of the risk of provoking uncontrolled hypercapnia. However, Strom and colleagues [23] have recently examined the role of domiciliary oxygen therapy in patients with severe thoracic spine deformities. In the group studied, almost 40% had additional pathology contributing to hypoxaemia (e.g. COPD, previous pulmonary tuberculosis). It seems that a proportion of patients with a significant component of ventilation–perfusion mismatch due to a combination of chest wall disease and parenchymal lung disease may benefit initially from oxygen therapy, although survival in patients over the age of 65 years was poor and a growing number of patients required home ventilation with time. These findings underline the importance of close monitoring of any hypercapnic patient receiving oxygen therapy. Overnight assessment of oximetry and transcutaneous CO_2 is strongly recommended.

Continuous positive airway pressure in respiratory failure

The use of CPAP in obstructive sleep apnoea in considered in Chapter 13. CPAP has been shown to reduce the work of breathing in COPD patients during exercise. It may also be of value in patients with respiratory decompensation due to a combination of obstructive sleep apnoea and COPD (overlap syndrome) of those in whom bulbar weakness outstrips general respiratory muscle weakness. However, in most patients with respiratory decompensation due to chest wall disease, neuromuscular conditions or COPD, CPAP is unable to offload respiratory muscles to the same extent as assisted ventilation, and does not control severe nocturnal hypoventilation.

Intermittent courses of non-invasive ventilation

A final strategy that may be employed before the introduction of home ventilation is intermittent courses of in-hospital non-invasive ventilation. Clearly this is of value in patients who develop an acute hypercapnic exacerbation of chronic lung disease, but occasionally patients who experience a gradual decline in ventilatory function may derive sustained improvement in arterial blood gas tensions and a reduction in symptoms after a short course of intensive nocturnal and diurnal NIPPV lasting approximately 7–10 days. Some of these patients may be maintained in good health by two or three courses of NIPPV a year (Fig. 7.3). The mechanism of action of this short period of treatment is under investigation, but it may work via a reduction in ventilatory load and 'resetting' of hypercapnic drive. Most patients initially maintained on intermittent courses of NIPPV will ultimately require domiciliary ventilation, although in-hospital courses of treatment may be helpful in individuals who cannot cope with ventilatory equipment in the home for social or practical reasons. It is also an economical use of often scarce equipment. Short course NIPPV should be distinguished from the practice of giving non-invasive ventilation on a regular weekly basis. This approach is controversial [24], and we have not found it helpful.

CRITERIA FOR STARTING DOMICILIARY VENTILATION

There are no hard and fast rules, but assuming all standard treatment has failed and the patient is motivated to try non-invasive ventilation, most authorities proceed to treatment in the presence of symptomatic diurnal

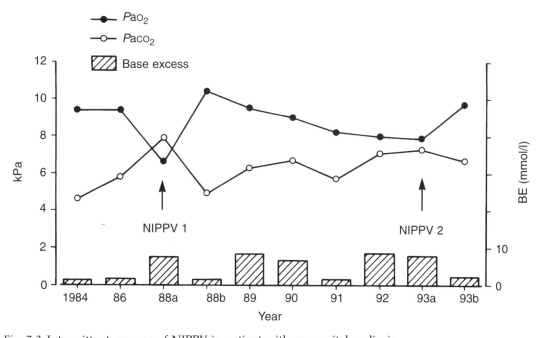

Fig. 7.3 Intermittent courses of NIPPV in patient with congenital scoliosis.

respiratory failure when mean overnight SaO_2 is less than 90% and PCO_2 exceeds 7 kPa. In severely hypercapnic patients with marked symptoms and stable underlying disease, the decision to start treatment is relatively easy. Recurrent admissions for acute hypercapnic exacerbation are also an important influencing factor. In those with milder, more intermittent symptoms a controlled trial to determine the optimum time for initiating therapy is probably indicated. At present there is *no* indication for NIPPV to be used prophylactically (i.e. before CO_2 retention has developed) in neuromuscular disease or any other disorder. Factors concerning choice of the method of ventilation are described in Chapter 3.

Familiarization with the technique during a brief hospital admission is advisable to address any initial teething problems, educate the patient and family, ensure the correct ventilatory settings, and instil confidence in all concerned. There is evidence to suggest that compliance with NIPPV is less good if treatment is started on an outpatient basis [25].

REFERENCES

1. Nachemson, A. (1968) A long term follow up study of non-treated kyphoscoliosis. *Acta Orthop. Scand.*, **39**, 466–76.
2. Freyschuss, V., Nilsonne, U. and Lundgren, K.D. (1968) Idiopathic scoliosis in old age. 1. Respiratory function. *Arch. Med. Scand.*, **184**: 365.
3. Branthwaite, M.A. (1986) Cardiorespiratory consequences of unfused idiopathic scoliosis. *Br. J. Dis. Chest*, **80**, 360–9.
4. Pehrsson, K., Bake, B., Larsson, S. and Nachemson, A. (1991) Lung function in adult idiopathic scoliosis: a 20 year follow-up. *Thorax*, **46**, 474–8.
5. Robert, D., Langevin, B. and Leger, P. (1991) Mouth leaks during non-invasive nasal intermittent positive pressure ventilation (Abstract). Proceedings 3rd Conference on Pulmonary Rehabilitation and Home Ventilation, Denver, 1991, p. 99.
6. Sawicka, E.H. and Branthwaite, M.A. (1987) Respiration during sleep in kyphoscoliosis. *Thorax*, **42**, 801–8.
7. Braun, N.M.T., Arora, N.S. and Rochester, D.F. (1983) Respiratory muscle and pulmonary function in polymyositis and other proximal myopathies. *Thorax*, **38**, 616–23.
8. Elliott, M.W. and Branthwaite, M.A. (1991) Occult respiratory failure as a cause of neuro-psychiatric symptoms in patients with chest wall deformity and neuromuscular disease. *Respir. Med.*, **85**, 431–3.
9. McLellan, P.A., Goldstein, R.S., Ramacharan, V. and Rebuck, A.S. (1981) Transcutaneous carbon dioxide monitoring. *Am. Rev. Respir. Dis.*, **124**, 199–201.
10. Sanders, M.H., Kern, N.B., Costantino, J.P. *et al.* (1994) Accuracy of end-tidal transcutaneous PCO_2 monitoring during sleep. *Chest*, **106**, 472–83.
11. Piper, A.J. and Sullivan, C.E. (1994) Breathing and neuromuscular disease, in *Sleep and Breathing* (eds N.A. Saunders and C.E. Sullivan). Marcel Dekker, New York, p. 777.
12. Green, M. and Moxham, J. (1993) Respiratory muscles in health and disease, in *Respiratory Medicine: Recent Advances* (ed. Peter J. Barnes), Butterworth-Heinemann, Oxford, pp. 252–75.
13. Simonds, A.K., Parker, R.A., Sawicka, E.H. and Branthwaite, M.A. (1986) Protriptyline for nocturnal hypoventilation in restrictive chest wall disease. *Thorax*, **41**, 586–90.
14. Carroll, N., Parker, R.A. and Branthwaite, M.A. (1990) The use of protriptyline for respiratory failure in patients with chronic airflow limitation. *Eur. Respir. J.*, **3**, 746–51.
15. Bonora, M., St John, W.M. and Bledsoe, T.A. (1985) Differential elevation by protriptyline and depression by diazepam of upper airway respiratory motor activity. *Am. Rev. Respir. Dis.*, **131**, 41–5.
16. Simonds, A.K., Carroll, N., Shiner, R. *et al.* (1988) Long term suppression of REM sleep in the treatment of sleep disordered breathing. *Thorax*, **43**, 851P.
17. Series, F., Cormier, M.Y. and La Forge, J. (1993) Long term effects of protriptyline in patients with chronic obstructive pulmonary disease. *Am. Rev. Respir. Dis.*, **147**, 1487–90.
18. Laubie, M. and Schmitt, H. (1980) Long lasting

hyperventilation induced by almitrine: evidence for a specific effect on carotid and thoracic chemoreceptors. *Eur. J. Pharmacol.*, **61**, 123–36.

19. Melot, C., Naerije, R., Rothschild, T. *et al.* (1983). Improvement in ventilation perfusion matching by almitrine. *Chest*, **83**, 528–33.

20. Skatrud, J.B., Dempsey, J.A., Iber, C. and Berssenbrugge, A. (1981) Correction of CO_2 retention during sleep in patients with chronic obstructive pulmonary disease. *Am. Rev. Respir. Dis.*, **124**, 260–8.

21. Skatrud, J.B. and Dempsey, J.A. (1983) Relative effectiveness of acetazolamide versus medroxyprogesterone acetate in correction of carbon dioxide retention. *Am. Rev. Respir. Dis.*, **127**, 405–12.

22. White, D.P., Zwillich, C.W., Pickett, C.K. *et al.* (1982) Central sleep apnea. Improvement with acetazolamide therapy. *Arch. Intern. Med.*, **142**, 1816–19.

23. Strom, K., Pehrsson, K., Boe, J. and Nachemson, A. (1992) Survival of patients with severe thoracic spine deformities receiving domiciliary oxygen therapy. *Chest*, **102**, 164–8.

24. Gutierrez, M., Beroiza, T., Contreras, G. *et al.* (1988) Weekly cuirass ventilation improves blood gases and inspiratory muscle strength in patients with chronic airflow limitation and hypercarbia. *Am. Rev. Respir. Dis.*, **138**, 617–23.

25. Elliott, M.W., Simonds, A.K., Carroll, M.P. *et al.* (1992) Domiciliary nocturnal nasal intermittent positive pressure ventilation in hypercapnic respiratory failure due to chronic obstructive lung disease: effects on sleep and quality of life. *Thorax*, **47**, 342–8.

8

Non-invasive ventilation in restrictive disorders and neuromuscular disease

ANITA K. SIMONDS

INTRODUCTION

In this chapter the evidence to support the use of non-invasive ventilation in restrictive disorders is presented, together with an analysis of outcome and discussion of the mechanisms of action. Most work has centred on the role of non-invasive ventilation in early onset idiopathic scoliosis, previous poliomyelitis, old tuberculous lung and chest wall disease and relatively stable muscular dystrophies and myopathies. The use of non-invasive ventilation during pregnancy in patients with scoliosis is also considered. Rapidly progressive neuromuscular disorders are covered in Chapters 11 and 12.

NEGATIVE PRESSURE VENTILATION IN RESTRICTIVE DISORDERS

Since the 1950s there have been numerous descriptive reports of the effects of negative pressure ventilation (nPV) in patients with scoliosis [1,2], thoracoplasty [3] and neuromuscular disease [4–6]. Much of this work dates from the renaissance of interest in nPV in the late 1970s and early 1980s. Splaingard et al. [4] have described 20 years' experience with domiciliary nPV in 40 patients with neuromuscular disease. The majority of patients were aged between 6 and 40 years and more than half had muscular dystrophy. Most used tank ventilators in the home, a few were ventilated with a cuirass or pneumosuit. Only three patients required supplemental oxygen therapy. Five-year and ten-year survival in this group was 76% and 61% respectively, despite 35% of patients having Duchenne muscular dystrophy. Three individuals required a tracheostomy for recurrent aspiration after several years of successful nPV. All patients were cared for at home by family members or volunteers. Equally instructive is a discussion in the same article of nine patients with neuromuscular disease in whom nPV was unsuccessful. Six of these subjects were under 3 years of age and experienced problems with recurrent aspiration and/or upper airway obstruction. Three older patients had a high cervico-thoracic scoliosis which caused problems obtaining a neck seal in the tank ventilator. Positive pressure ventilation via tracheostomy was effective in most of these technical nPV failures. The authors summarize their work over the period 1962–1982, and it is likely that NIPPV would now be used for at least some of the older patients without bulbar problems in whom nPV was unsuccessful.

Non-Invasive Respiratory Support. Edited by Anita Simonds. Published by Chapman & Hall, London. ISBN 0412 56840 3.

A variety of negative pressure techniques (including cuirass, tank ventilator, pneumojacket and pneumobody suit) were used by Sawicka and colleagues [7] in an analysis of outcome in 51 patients with restrictive disorders (5 progressive neuromuscular disease, 24 slowly progressive or static neuromuscular disease and 22 with skeletal deformity). Improvement in exercise tolerance and reduction in breathlessness was seen in all patients, accompanied by a significant increase in PaO_2 and $PaCO_2$. Around 20% of patients developed upper airway obstruction during sleep which limited the efficiency of nPV and was treated with either protriptyline or tracheostomy. Other workers have treated nPV-induced upper airway obstruction during sleep with CPAP [2], although a switch to NIPPV is now regarded as simpler and more logical.

Upper airway obstruction is reported to be the commonest cause of desaturation during sleep with nPV and occurs in both patients and control subjects [2,8]. These obstructive episodes can result in arousals, and are caused by the failure of normal inspiratory activation of the upper airway abductors. Diaphragm and upper airway muscle function are therefore uncoordinated leading to upper airway collapse. The frequency of upper airway obstruction during nPV appears to be higher in males.

NIPPV IN RESTRICTIVE DISORDERS

As with nPV, the effectiveness of NIPPV was first explored in patients with neuromuscular disease and chest wall disorders [9–11]. Delaubier and Rideau were the earliest exponents of its use in patients with Duchenne muscular dystrophy [12]. With the rapid uptake of the technique a substantial database has accumulated over the past 5–8 years. However, as NIPPV only entered widespread clinical practice in 1986/7, long-term outcome information is limited.

In a large French multicentre series [13] of 276 patents receiving domiciliary NIPPV, the greatest overall improvement was seen in patients with scoliosis and post-tuberculous sequelae. Over a 3-year period 27% of patients discontinued NIPPV. Only a minority of patients stopped treatment voluntarily (5% of restrictive patients compared to 11% of COPD patients). Fifteen per cent of the scoliotic and post-tuberculous patients died, with most deaths due to respiratory problems; 6% were transferred to tracheostomy-IPPV (T-IPPV).

The 5-year actuarial probability of continuing domiciliary NIPPV in 180 patients from a single centre in the United Kingdom was 79% (95% CI, 66–92) for scoliotic patients, 100% in post-poliomyelitis patients, 94% (95%, CI 83–100) in post-tuberculous cases, 81% (95%, CI, 61–100) in those with neuromuscular disorders excluding poliomyelitis, compared to 43% (95% CI, 6–80) in COPD patients and less than 20% in individuals with bronchiectasis (see Fig. 8.1). The probability of continuing NIPPV closely approximates survival as death was the main cause of discontinuing NIPPV in this series. No patient was transferred to T-IPPV. Reasons for withdrawal of NIPPV and causes of death in patients with restrictive disorders compared to those with obstructive ventilatory disease are given in Table 8.1. Deaths in the restrictive group were due to either concurrent disease or cardiorespiratory failure in those with progressive neuromuscular disease or individuals who had been referred late for treatment.

EFFECTS OF NON-INVASIVE VENTILATION ON PHYSIOLOGICAL MEASURES

nPV

Sustained improvements in diurnal arterial blood gas tensions have been consistently

71

Restrictive disorders and neuromuscular disease

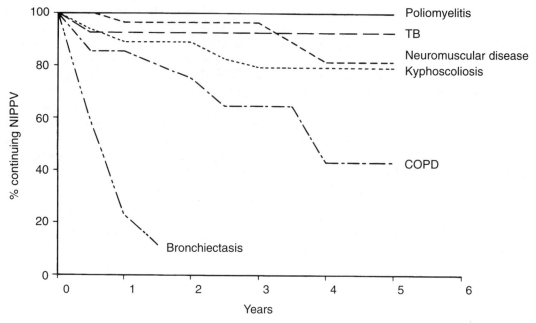

Fig. 8.1 Five-year probability of continuing NIPPV in patients with restrictive and obstructive disorders.

Table 8.1 Duration of NIPPV and reasons for withdrawal

	Median (range) duration of NIPPV (yr)	*Reasons for withdrawal*
Early onset scoliosis (*n* = 47)	3.2 (0.1–6.9)	Died 7 (5 respiratory failure, 1 carcinoma breast 1 carcinoma ovary) Discontinued 1 – improved
Previous polio (*n* = 30)	4.3 (0.6–6.4)	No withdrawals
Previous tuberculosis (*n* = 20)	2.1 (0.1–7)	Died 1 (leukaemia)
Neuromuscular disorders (*n* = 29)	2.8 (0.3–5.9)	Died 4 (respiratory failure due to progression of underlying disorder
COPD (*n* = 33)	1.6 (0.1–6.3)	Died 6 (respiratory failure) Withdrawn 5 – poor tolerance NIPPV
Bronchiectasis (*n* = 13)	0.7 (0.1–2.3)	Died 7 (respiratory failure) Withdrawn 2 – heart/lung transplantation
Miscellaneous (*n* = 8)	1.6 (0.2–4.8)	Died 1 (respiratory failure)

Source: Simonds and Elliott, 1995 [19].

demonstrated in restrictive patients using nPV predominantly during sleep. Hill [14] has summarized the outcome from a number of studies and shown that following nocturnal nPV, mean PaO_2 rose from 6.7 to 9.2 kPa and $PaCO_2$ fell from 8.8 to 6.1 kPa. Almost identical results were seen in the patients of Sawicka *et al.* [7]. This improvement in arterial blood gas tensions occurs rapidly. In 20 patients receiving nPV 16 hours/day maximum changes in blood gases were obtained after 12 weeks

(Fig. 8.2). Base excess fell in this group from 7.4 mmol/l to 1.9 mmol/l. It may be that intensive corrective non-invasive ventilation should be continued until base excess is normalized. In this group vital capacity rose significantly from a pre-treatment level of 750 ml (range 200–1150 ml) to 960 ml (range 350–1700 ml). As a percentage of predicted vital capacity the increase from 21.3 to 26.7% is less impressive.

A similar increase in vital capacity in re-

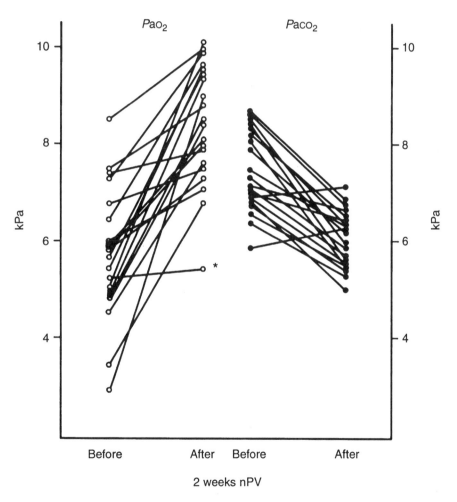

Fig. 8.2 Effect of negative pressure ventilation on ambulant arterial blood gas tensions in restrictive chest wall patients receiving 16 hours nPV in a tank ventilator per day. (*Patient also had cyanotic congenital heart disease).

strictive patients has been seen in other uncontrolled studies. Rochester, Braun and colleagues [15] were among the first to attribute changes in lung function to an increase in respiratory muscle strength occasioned by 'resting' the muscles during assisted ventilation. This theory is based on the hypothesis that respiratory muscle fatigue is a major factor in the development of ventilatory failure (Chapter 2). Certainly a decrease in integrated electromyogram activity (EMG) emanating from the diaphragm, intercostal and accessory muscles can be demonstrated during nPV [16] and NIPPV [17] (Fig. 8.3). In one study [15] diaphragm activity in a tank ventilator fell to 9% of the level when the subject was spontaneously breathing. Decreases in respiratory muscle activity may be even more marked during NIPPV. Increases in global respiratory muscle strength have been demonstrated in some studies, although findings are not consistent. In one series [18] maximum inspiratory mouth pressure rose from 27 to 43 cmH$_2$O and maximum expiratory mouth pressure increased from 58 to 73 cmH$_2$O. There was no correlation between the gain in respiratory muscle strength and changes in arterial blood gas tensions. It is possible that in these uncontrolled studies the improvement in respiratory muscle strength is at least in part due to increased motivation associated with better blood gases and sense of well-being. As a consequence the role of respiratory muscle rest in restrictive disorders is unclear, but it is of interest that when an increase in respiratory muscle strength is seen it often occurs within hours of initiating assisted ventilation before significant changes in ambulant arterial blood gas tensions have occurred. These data contrast with the findings in COPD patients where increases in respiratory muscle strength are not seen (Chapter 9).

In terms of functional outcome 46% of patients receiving nPV for stable or slowly progressive neuromuscular disorders returned to work and 71% of those with skeletal deformities were in employment at the time of follow-up [7]. Although relief of symptoms was seen in patients with progressive disorders, all continued to deteriorate and died from cardiorespiratory failure a median of 13 months (range 3–27 months) after starting treatment.

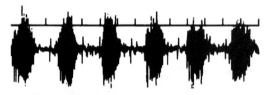

Spontaneous ventilation

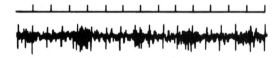

In tank 5 min

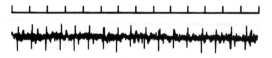

In tank 30 min

Fig. 8.3 Reduction in diaphragmatic surface electromyogram in patient starting negative pressure ventilation.

NIPPV

In patients with restrictive disorders, improvements in arterial blood gas tensions are comparable if not superior to those obtained with nPV (Fig. 8.4).

The outcome from the UK series [19] closely

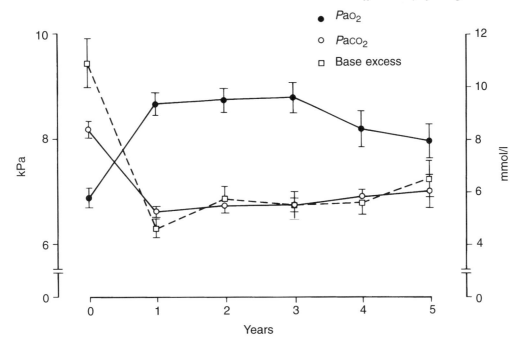

Fig. 8.4 Effect of long-term domicilliary NIPPV in restrictive ventilatory disorders. Reproduced from Simonds and Elliot [19].

matches that of the French study [13], despite the fact that the UK patients were more hypoxaemic and hypercapnic on starting NIPPV, and used less supplemental oxygen than the French patients (e.g. 60% of French scoliosis patients received O_2 with NIPPV, compared to 8.5% of UK patients).

A further improvement in PaO_2 and $PaCO_2$ can be demonstrated in transferring restrictive patients from nPV to NIPPV (Fig. 8.5). This is likely to be due to a lesser tendency to upper airway obstruction during sleep and the greater mechanical efficiency of NIPPV. NIPPV is also more effective than nPV in younger patients [20] and individuals with Duchenne muscular dystrophy [6], especially those who are shown to have concurrent obstructive sleep apnoea. In contrast to this, Jackson *et al.* [21] have reported comparable outcome in two groups with restrictive disorders matched for age, sex and primary diagnosis treated with nPV or NIPPV. How-

ever, treatment was not randomized and PaO_2 at the start of treatment appeared lower in the NIPPV group.

Vital capacity has not been shown to change significantly during 5 years of NIPPV [13,19], although anecdotal reports indicate an early increase in lung volumes can be seen. There is little information on the long-term effects of NIPPV on muscle function. An increase in hypercapnic drive would be expected as a result of reducing chronic hypercapnia and base excess. Improved sleep quality is also reported, which may further improve ventilatory drive and arousal reflex, although this has not been confirmed.

Chest wall compliance tends to be reduced in patients with restrictive disorders and it has been hypothesized that the regular stretching action of NIPPV may improve chest wall (+/− pulmonary) compliance. Conflicting evidence exists on this score [22–24].

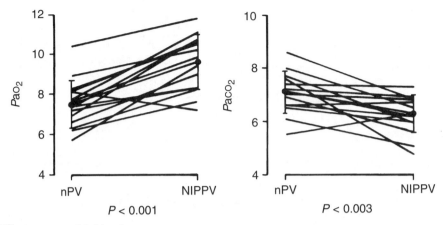

Fig. 8.5 Effect on arterial blood gas tensions of changing from nPV to NIPPV in 15 patients with restrictive disorders.

QUALITY OF LIFE AND HEALTH STATUS

All assessments of the impact of a treatment for a chronic disorder should take into account its effects on quality of life as well as morbidity and mortality. This is overwhelmingly important in patients with progressive disorders in whom the treatment may not affect the natural history of the condition. There are a number of tools designed to measure generic and specific aspects of the quality of life. Not all have been validated in the heterogenous group of patients who have been treated with NIPPV, so that results and especially comparisons with other treatments should be treated with caution.

However, a Swedish group [25] has examined overall health status using the Sickness Impact Profile (SIP) and Hospital Anxiety and Depression scale. Of a total of 39 patients with restrictive disorders receiving home ventilation, 29 received NIPPV. Psychosocial functioning and mental well-being was equally good in patients and a control group, despite lower indices of physical function in the patients. Sleep quality was reported as generally good. Of note is the fact that the

global quality of life estimation was mainly determined by the mental state of the patients and their sleep quality, with physical function having little influence. Patients with scoliosis scored higher on quality of life measures than patients with neuromuscular disease. Interestingly, low standard bicarbonate levels and $PaCO_2$ were correlated with higher levels of mental well-being. Health status in patients recieving T-IPPV did not differ from those using NIPPV in this study. Other work has shown, however, that non-invasive methods of ventilation are preferable to both patients and carers [26].

In the French series a comparison of hospital admissions during the year before initiation of NIPPV and the year following showed a significant decrease [13]. In the scoliotic group 34 days were spent in hospital before NIPPV, compared to 6 days when receiving NIPPV. A majority of patients reported improvement in sleep quality (62%) and an increase in their ability to carry out activities of daily living (70%).

In the UK study [19], the SF-36 self-administered questionnaire was used in a cross-section of 116 domiciliary NIPPV recipients with an average age of 54 years. The SF-36 is a measure of general health status which assesses physical function, role limitation due to physical or mental problems, social function, mental health, energy and vitality, pain and health perception [27,28]. The response rate was 90.5%. Physical function was significantly higher in the patients with idiopathic scoliosis, and those with post-poliomyelitis and post-tuberculous disease compared to the group with neuromuscular disorders and obstructive lung disease. It is noteworthy that the neuromuscular group (containing those with progressive muscular dystrophies) and the COPD group had similar scores for physical function, but perceived role limitation due to physical factors was greater in the COPD patients. Health status in NIPPV recipients as a whole was comparable to that in a study of ambulant outpatients in the USA with chronic disorders such as cardiac failure. Unsurprisingly, physical function was reduced compared to age-matched 'normals' recruited in a general practice study, but, as with the Swedish study, scores for mental health and energy and vitality were similar.

These results contradict the commonly held belief that ventilator-dependent patients have a poor quality of life and are severely limited in functional terms.

MECHANISMS OF ACTION OF NON-INVASIVE VENTILATION IN RESTRICTIVE DISORDERS

As indicated above, relief of respiratory muscle fatigue, an improvement in chest wall compliance and control of nocturnal hypoventilation have all been postulated as the mechanism by which diurnal blood gas tensions are corrected long term in patients receiving non-invasive ventilation. Of course, none of these are mutually exclusive, and in different pathologies at different times all may play a part. Although few studies of

ventilatory drive have been carried out, currently the most persuasive theory is that benefit is derived by the correction of arterial blood gas tensions overnight resulting in enhanced ventilatory drive and better quality sleep.

In support of this conclusion are the results for a study carried out by Hill *et al.* [29]. Here the efficacy of nocturnal NIPPV was examined by withholding treatment in restrictive patients who were well acclimatized to NIPPV. All patients had demonstrated an improvement in symptoms and arterial blood gas tensions on NIPPV. A week after withdrawal patients experienced more breathlessness, morning headaches, somnolence and less energ in *the absence* of any change in daytime arterial blood gas tensions, pulmonary function or respiratory muscle strength. However, nocturnal monitoring off NIPPV showed a greater degree of tachycardia and tachypnoea, more desaturation and a larger rise in $Paco_2$ than on NIPPV, indicating that control of nocturnal hypoventilation is an important feature of NIPPV.

PREGNANCY AND SCOLIOSIS

In scoliotic patients the physiological changes associated with pregnancy, including an increase in minute ventilation by 40%, a reduction in functional residual capacity and rise in cardiac output by around 2.5 l/minute, can pose problems. Progression of the spinal curvature may occur and flaring of the lower ribs caused by the expanding uterus can cause long-term mechanical difficulties [30], although this is rare. In spite of these risks, pregnancy in patients with idiopathic scoliosis is often tolerated remarkably well [31,32]. Contraindications to pregnancy are the presence of established pulmonary hypertension and hypoxaemia [33]. Individuals with a vital capacity of less than 1 litre are at high risk [30]. Pre-pregnancy counselling is vital to assess the hazards for the mother and fetus,

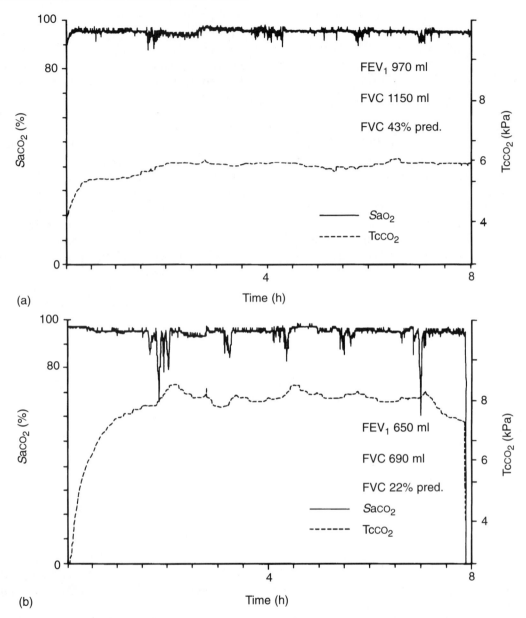

Fig. 8.6 Spirometry and overnight monitoring of arterial oxygen saturation and transcutaneous CO_2 in (a) patient with congenital scoliosis who underwent an uneventful pregnancy and (b) patient with congenital scoliosis who developed cor pumonale near term during an unplanned pregnancy.

and also to evaluate genetic and obstetric risks. A full assessment should include ECG, echocardiogram, measurement of lung func-tion and arterial blood gases, and monitoring of respiration during sleep if nocturnal hypoventilation is suspected. Figure 8.6

shows overnight monitoring of arterial oxygen saturation (Sa_{O_2}), Tc_{CO_2}, plus spirometry in two females with congenital idiopathic scoliosis: (a) underwent an uneventful pregnancy but (b) developed cor pulmonale at 36 weeks during an unplanned pregnancy. Note the presence of a vital capacity less than 1 litre and significant nocturnal hypoventilation in (b).

Patients who present *de novo* to the respiratory physician with respiratory failure and cor pulmonale at an advanced stage of pregnancy pose a difficult problem. It is important to avoid the misdiagnosis of pre-eclampsia in this situation. Negative pressure ventilation has been used successfully to salvage both mother and baby [30], and may avert premature labour. It seems likely that NIPPV is equally effective, and easier to apply [34].

CONCLUSIONS

There has been no controlled trial of nPV or NIPPV in restrictive disorders. However, the literature abounds with reports demonstrating a positive outcome. Although a bias towards publishing positive results may play a part, the overwhelming evidence supports the use of non-invasive ventilation in these patients, so that a controlled trial with one group of patients randomized not to receive non-invasive ventilation is probably unethical. NIPPV is usually superior to nPV, but comparable results may be achieved in some patient groups.

REFERENCES

1. Garay, S.M., Turino, G.M. and Goldring, R.M. (1981) Sustained reversal of chronic hypercapnia in patients with alveolar hypoventilation syndromes. *Am. J. Med.*, **70**, 269–74.
2. Goldstein, R.S., Molotiu, N., Skrastins, R. et al. (1987) Reversal of sleep-induced hypoventilation and chronic respiratory failure by nocturnal negative pressure ventilation in patients with restrictive ventilatory impairment. *Am. Rev. Respir. Dis.*, **135**, 1049–55.
3. Sawicka, E.H., Branthwaite, M.A. and Spencer, G.T. (1983) Respiratory failure after thoracoplasty: treatment by intermittent negative pressure ventilation. *Thorax*, **38**, 433–5.
4. Splaingard, M.L., Jefferson, L.S. and Harrison, G.M. (1982) Survival of patients with respiratory insufficiency secondary to neuromuscular disease treated at home with negative pressure ventilation (Abstract). *Am. Rev. Respir. Dis.*, **125**, 139.
5. Mohr, C.H. and Hill, N.S. (1990) Long-term follow-up of nocturnal ventilatory assistance in patients with respiratory failure due to Duchenne-type muscular dystrophy. *Chest*, **97**, 91–6.
6. Hill, N.S., Redline, S., Carskadon, M. et al. (1992) Sleep-disordered breathing in patients with Duchenne muscular dystrophy using negative pressure ventilators. *Chest*, **102**, 1656–62.
7. Sawicka, E.H., Loh, L. and Branthwaite, M.A. (1988) Domicilary ventilatory support; an analysis of outcome. *Thorax*, **43**, 31–5.
8. Levy, R.D., Bradley, T.D., Newman, S.L. et al. (1989) Negative pressure ventilation: effects on ventilation during sleep in normal subjects. *Chest*, **95**, 95–9.
9. Leger, P., Jennequin, J., Gerard, M., et al. (1989) Home positive pressure ventilation via nasal mask for patients with neuromusculoskeletal disorders. *Eur. Respir. J.*, **2**(Suppl. 7), 640s–5s.
10. Kerby, G.R., Mayer, L.S. and Pingleton, S.K. (1987) Nocturnal positive pressure ventilation via nasal mask. *Am. Rev. Respir. Dis.*, **135**, 738–40.
11. Carroll, N. and Branthwaite, M.A. (1988) Control of nocturnal hypoventilation by nasal intermittent positive pressure ventilation. *Thorax*, **43**, 349–53.
12. Rideau, Y. and Delaubier, A. (1988) Management of respiratory neuromuscular weakness. *Muscle and Nerve*, **11**, 407–8.
13. Leger, P., Bedicam, J.M., Cornette, A. et al. (1994) Nasal intermittent positive pressure

ventilation. Long term follow-up in patients with severe chronic respiratory insufficiency. *Chest*, **105**, 100–5.

14. Hill, N. (1993) Noninvasive ventilation. Does it work, for whom, and how? *Am. Rev. Respir. Dis.*, **147**, 1050–5.

15. Rochester, D.F., Braun, N.M. and Laine, S. (1977) Diaphragmatic energy expenditure in chronic respiratory failure. *Am. J. Med.*, **63**, 223–31.

16. Marino, W. and Braun, N.M.T. (1982) Reversal of the clinical sequelae of respiratory muscle fatigue by intermittent mechanical ventilation. *Am. Rev. Respir. Dis.*, **125**, 85.

17. Carrey, Z., Gottfried, S.B. and Levy R.D. (1990) Ventilatory muscle support in respiratory failure with nasal positive pressure ventilation. *Chest*, **97**, 150–8.

18. Simonds, A.K. (1987) The management of alveolar hypoventilation in restrictive chest wall disease. MD Thesis, University of London.

19. Simonds, A.K. and Elliott, M.W. (1995) Outcome of domiciliary nasal intermittent positive pressure ventilation. *Thorax*, **50**, 604–9.

20. Heckmatt, J.Z., Loh, L. and Dubowitz, V. (1990) Night-time nasal ventilation in neuromuscular disease. *Lancet*, **335**, 579–82.

21. Jackson, M., Hockley, S., King, M.A. and Shneerson, J.M. (1991) A comparison of the physiological results of treatment with NIPPV or cuirass ventilation (Abstract). *Am. Rev. Respir. Dis.*, **143**, A585.

22. Sinha, R. and Bergofsky, E.H. (1972) Prolonged alteration of lung mechanics in kyphoscoliosis by positive pressure hyperinflation. *Am. Rev. Respir. Dis.*, **106**, 47–57.

23. De Troyer, A. and Deisser, P. (1981) The effects of intermittent positive pressure breathing on patients with respiratory muscle weakness. *Am. Rev. Respir. Dis.*, **124**, 132–7.

24. Simonds, A.K., Parker, R.A. and Branthwaite, M.A. (1989) The effect of intermittent positive-pressure hyperinflation in restrictive chest wall disease. *Respiration*, **55**, 136–43.

25. Pehrsson, K., Olofson, J., Larsson, S. and Sullivan, M. (1994) Quality of life in patients treated by home mechanical ventilation due to restrictive ventilatory disorders. *Respir. Med.*, **88**, 21–6.

26. Bach, J. (1993) A comparison of long-term ventilatory support alternatives from the perspective of the patient and care-giver. *Chest*, **104**, 1702–6.

27. Ware, J.E. (1993) Measuring patients' views: the optimum outcome measure. SF-36: a valid, reliable assessment of health from a patient's point of view. *Br. Med. J.*, **306**, 1429–30.

28. Brazier, J.E., Harper, R., Jones, N.M.B. *et al.* (1992) Validating the SF-36 health survey questionnaire: new outcome measure for primary care. *Br. Med. J.*, **305**, 160–4.

29. Hill, N.S., Eveloff, S.E., Carlisle, C.C. and Goff, S.G. (1992) Efficacy of nocturnal nasal ventilation in patients with restrictive thoracic disease. *Am. Rev. Respir. Dis.*, **145**, 365–71.

30. Sawicka, E.H., Spencer, G.T. and Branthwaite, M.A. (1986) Management of respiratory failure complicating pregnancy in severe kyphoscoliosis: a new use for an old technique? *Br. J. Dis. Chest*, **80**, 191–6.

31. Manning, C.W., Prime, F.J. and Zorab, P.A. (1967) Pregnancy and scoliosis. *Lancet*, **2**, 792–5.

32. Siegler, D. and Zorab, P.A. (1981) Pregnancy in thoracic scoliosis. *Br. J. Dis. Chest*, **75**, 367–70.

33. De Swiet, M. (1987) Chest diseases in pregnancy, in *Oxford Texbook of Medicine* (eds D.J. Weatherall, J.G.G. Ledingham and D.A. Warrell). Oxford Medical Publications, Oxford, pp. 27–9.

34. Gaucherand, P., Gerard, M., Prud'hon, M.C., Gelas, M., Robert, D. and Rudigoz, R.C. (1990) Chronic and severe respiratory insufficiency and pregnancy. A new way to treating it. *Journal de Gynaecologie, Obstetrique et Biologie de la Reproduction*, **19**(2), 197–201.

9

Non-invasive ventilation in chronic obstructive pulmonary disease

MARK W. ELLIOTT

INTRODUCTION

Long-term oxygen therapy (LTOT) is the only therapy which has been shown to improve survival in patients with respiratory failure because of chronic obstructive pulmonary disease (COPD) [1,2]. It is the first line treatment for such patients, but it is reasonable to continue to explore alternatives. First, although compliance with LTOT was very good in the trials this is not always the case in routine clinical practice, the main reason being the restriction placed upon lifestyle by the need for 15 hours' oxygen per day. Symptomatic patients who gain subjective benefit from LTOT are more likely to comply with therapy, but asymptomatic patients tend to use oxygen for insufficient time to gain survival benefit [3,4]. Secondly, an interesting finding in the Medical Research Council (MRC) trial was that no survival advantage from oxygen became apparent until 500 days' treatment had elapsed. The best predictor of death, and therefore a lack of benefit from oxygen, during this period was a combination of polycythaemia and hypercapnia. The Nocturnal Oxygen therapy trial (NOTT) study showed that a change in haematocrit was unrelated to survival and this therefore suggests that hypercapnia may be responsible for the worse prognosis and lack of response to oxygen therapy. Further evidence for this hypothesis comes from the study of Cooper et al. [5] in which, although the benefit from oxygen was apparent immediately, 29 of the 57 patients who were hypercapnic at entry, died during the course of the study compared with only three of 15 normocapnic patients.

The reason why hypercapnia should be associated with a worse prognosis is not clear. Death occurs more often at night in patients with COPD than in age-matched controls and is most likely in those with hypoxaemia and hypercapnia [6]. Severe oxygen desaturation is more likely during sleep in patients who are hypercapnic by day and it is therefore possible that the worse response to oxygen in hypercapnic patients was a consequence of a failure to abolish severe episodes of nocturnal oxygen desaturation. In both the MRC and NOTT studies death often occurred at night, sometimes with a history of increasing respiratory difficulty. However, it is important not to equate nocturnal death with death during sleep. In the NOTT study patients were given sufficient oxygen to increase PaO_2 into the

Non-Invasive Respiratory Support. Edited by Anita Simonds. Published by Chapman & Hall, London. ISBN 0412 56840 3.

range 60–80 mmHg while awake and were told to increase the flow rate by 1 l/min during exercise and sleep. In the MRC study the same criteria were used during wakefulness but no changes to flow rate were made during sleep and it is therefore possible that severe oxygen desaturation was not eliminated in the hypercapnic patients. It is interesting to speculate that if the oxygen flow rate had also been increased during sleep in the British patients, improvement in survival might have been seen immediately. However, high flow oxygen therapy may cause worsening CO_2 retention and acidosis, which in turn may be detrimental.

The effect of the interaction between hypoxia and hypercapnia upon the human pulmonary circulation is not well known. However, in isolated animal preparations hypercapnia, in the presence of hypoxia, leads to a variety of different responses in the pulmonary circulation; vasoconstriction (dogs), vasodilatation (rats) or a biphasic response (cats) [7]. In man acidosis is a potent vasoconstrictor and therefore transient rises in CO_2 during sleep may exacerbate the vasoconstrictor response to hypoxia. There may therefore be advantages, in terms of pulmonary haemodynamics, if hypercapnia is improved as well as hypoxia.

Impaired sleep quality is well recognized in COPD compared to age-matched controls [8] and experience from patients with obstructive sleep apnoea (OSA) suggests that sleep disruption is associated with impaired neuropsychiatric functioning and reduced quality of life [9]. The effect of oxygen on sleep quality is contentious, with some investigators showing an improvement [10] and others no benefit [11]. CO_2 tension was not measured in either of these studies and although severe hypoxia ($Sao_2 < 70\%$) may not cause arousal in humans [12], acute hypercapnia, with a rise in $Paco_2$ of 6–15 mmHg, has been shown to be a reliable and powerful arousal stimulus [13]. Alterna-

tively, sleep quality may be impaired by increased respiratory effort, as seen in patients with increased upper airway resistance [14], because of loading of respiratory muscles. Therefore, assisted ventilation may improve sleep quality by reducing carbon dioxide or unloading respiratory muscles.

In patients with extrapulmonary restrictive disorders overnight CO_2 tensions are improved, as are diurnal blood gas tensions, when ventilation is assisted mechanically during sleep alone, leaving the patient free to pursue normal activities during the day. Its use during sleep alone in patients with COPD may therefore circumvent some of the problems of LTOT and may improve survival. The possible advantages of mechanically assisted ventilation over LTOT in COPD can be summarized as follows:

- improved compliance (?);
- improved survival (?);
- improved sleep quality (?)
  because of reduced CO_2
  because of unloading of respiratory muscles.

MECHANICALLY ASSISTED VENTILATION IN COPD

The concept of mechanically assisted ventilation in COPD is not new. It was first tried by day using **intermittent positive pressure breathing** (IPPB) through a mouthpiece. The technique involves active inflation of the lungs under positive pressure and of passive deflation during expiration, primarily produced by the elastic recoil of the lungs and the chest wall. Gas flow from the machine ceases when a predetermined pressure is reached, and the expiratory pathway is then open to atmosphere. Machines in use today, primarily as a physiotherapy adjunct, include the Bird (M and IE Dentsply, Sowton Industrial Estate, Exeter) and the Bennett (UK supplier: Puritan Bennett, 152–176 Great South West Road, Hounslow, Middlesex).

IPPB has been shown to reduce $PaCO_2$ [15] or abolish the rise of $PaCO_2$ associated with breathing 100% O_2 [16]. This is usually the result of an increase in tidal volume (V_T), and hence increase in MV and fall in the ratio of dead space to V_T. It has been said to decrease the work and oxygen cost of breathing [15,17], but both of these claims have been disputed [18,19]. There are no data about its use during sleep.

Studies of the chronic use of IPPB in COPD have shown no consistent benefit [20–23]. In the largest study, 985 patients were randomized to IPPB or conventional therapy [23]. In the treatment group patients were asked to use IPPB for 10 minutes three times a day during which time they inhaled a beta agonist generated by the machine's nebulizer. The control group had the same treatment administered by compressor over the same time. There were no statistically significant differences in mortality, need for hospitalization, change in lung function or quality of life during an average follow-up of 33 months. The main conclusion was that IPPB was no better than a compressor in providing nebulized bronchodilators. However, in all the studies the duration of each treatment session was no more than 20 minutes, which is unlikely to be long enough to have a lasting physiological effect. Because the inspiratory phase is terminated as soon as the predetermined pressure is reached, it is unlikely that these machines will provide effective ventilation in most patients with COPD in whom the impedance to inflation is high and may change with time.

NEGATIVE PRESSURE VENTILATION

Various trials of in-hospital assisted ventilation, using negative pressure devices, in patients with COPD have been reported [24–28]. Ventilation has usually been assisted during wakefulness with the aim of reducing respiratory muscle activity and allowing recovery from 'respiratory muscle fatigue'. In these uncontrolled studies improvements, sometimes striking, in a variety of variables have been attributed to relatively short periods of assisted ventilation. In many patients it is possible that the improvements seen simply reflected the natural recovery from an acute exacerbation.

Attempts at using negative pressure ventilators during sleep or at home have not been successful [28–30]. In the study of Zibrak and colleagues [29], only nine of 20 patients enrolled in a crossover study, comparing domiciliary nPV using a ponchowrap ventilator with conventional treatment, completed both 6-month periods of the trial. All but one of the patients who completed the study expressed dissatisfaction, using the equipment for an average of 4 hours per day instead of the 16 hours a day that had been recommended. Despite continued encouragement none of the patients could sleep with the ventilator, because of discomfort. Inadequate ventilation during sleep with negative pressure devices may be a particular problem because of the development of upper airway obstruction [8,31–33]. After 3–6 months nPV there was no clinically significant difference in lung function, daytime arterial blood gas tensions or exercise capacity.

In another in-hospital study, with a control group who received standard pulmonary rehabilitation [28], patients who received nPV were unable to sleep with the equipment and used it considerably less than advised during the day. Fourteen patients completed the study and there was no difference between the two groups, with both showing clinical improvement and an increase in exercise tolerance. Following the trial, of 8 patients randomized to nPV who completed the study, one did not want to take the ventilator home and four discontinued treatment within 3 months because of a lack of any perceived benefit. Only one patient continued nPV at 2 years.

In a large controlled study of 184 patients with COPD randomized to either active or sham nPV at home [30], 10 patients did not use the respirators at home at all and 53 stopped treatment before the 12-week study period was complete. The main reasons for stopping were hospital admission ($n = 17$) and difficulties with the technique, including discomfort ($n = 24$). Patients were unable to use the ventilators during sleep and the mean daily use was only 3.5 hours. There were no statistically significant differences in exercise capacity, daytime arterial blood gas tensions, severity of dyspnoea, quality of life or respiratory muscle strength.

The conclusions from these studies are that negative pressure ventilation at home in patients with COPD is poorly tolerated, cannot be administered during sleep and results in little benefit.

POSITIVE PRESSURE VENTILATION VIA TRACHEOSTOMY

In a retrospective study, survival in 50 COPD patients ventilated at home via a tracheostomy [34] was little different from oxygen-treated patients in the MRC study of long-term oxygen therapy [1]. However, survival was no worse, despite the presence of a tracheostomy, which may be associated with a significant morbidity and mortality [35]. Additionally, patients were ventilated when the PaO_2 was less than 50 mmHg, but without apparent regard to the $PaCO_2$. In all studies of assisted ventilation in COPD, including those which have shown no overall benefit, it is clear that it is hypercapnic patients who are most likely to benefit. Hypoxia without hypercapnia is not unusual in COPD and it is likely that the patient group included patients without significant hypercapnia, who are less likely to benefit from ventilatory assistance.

Another retrospective study of 259 COPD patients ventilated at home via tracheostomy showed similar results, but survival was better than the oxygen-treated patients in the MRC study, until the fourth year when the survival curves rejoined [36]. Comparisons of prospective and retrospective trials should be made with caution, however overall it can be concluded that domiciliary positive pressure ventilation via tracheostomy is feasible, but the invasive nature is a significant disincentive to this approach.

NASAL INTERMITTENT POSITIVE PRESSURE VENTILATION

NIPPV avoids some of the disadvantages associated with both nPV and tracheostomy and has been used at home during sleep in COPD patients with some success. Carroll and Branthwaite [31] included four patients with COPD who benefited from NIPPV, albeit to a lesser extent than in those with extrapulmonary restrictive disease. Marino [37] showed reduced respiratory rate (29 ± 4 to 20 ± 4/min), $PaCO_2$ (67 ± 8 to 49 ± 9 mmHg) and heart rate (111 ± 15 to 81 ± 10/min) in nine (eight with COPD) out of 13 patients with progressive chronic ventilatory failure when started on NIPPV in hospital. Of the eight patients with COPD, four found the system so uncomfortable that they did not wish to continue, but the remaining four continued using the ventilator at home daily for periods of 6–10 months. They had improved physical capacity and daytime $PaCO_2$ at follow-up (mean 20 months).

In a study [38] with negative results, 19 patients with severe COPD took part in a randomized crossover trial of conventional treatment versus NIPPV during sleep using the BiPAP ventilator (Respironics Inc., Murrysville, Pennsylvania, USA). Seven patients withdrew because of intolerance of the nasal mask and five because of intercurrent illness. Seven patients completed both arms of the study, using the machine for a mean of 6.7 hours each night. There were no differences in any measured variable between the two treatments, except for improved neuropsychological performance following NIPPV.

In contrast to these results, Elliott *et al.* [39] showed some improvement in eight of twelve patients with COPD and hypercapnic ventilatory failure receiving NIPPV at home during sleep. At 6 months eight were continuing with NIPPV. One patient had died and three had withdrawn because they were unable to sleep with the equipment. Full polysomnography performed during NIPPV in patients continuing treatment at 6 months showed an increase in mean arterial oxygen saturation (SaO_2) of 11% (+2 to +23%), $P < 0.05$, and lower mean $TcCO_2$ -2.7 kPa (-1.3 to -5.1), $P < 0.05$, overnight compared with spontaneous breathing before starting NIPPV. Total sleep time increased during NIPPV by +72.5 minutes (+21 to +204 minutes), $P < 0.05$, but sleep architecture and the number of arousals were unchanged. Quality of life did not change, but was no worse during NIPPV. Six patients showed a reduction and two an increase in $PaCO_2$, median (range) for eight patients -0.9 kPa (-1.5 to $+0.4$), $P < 0.05$, and seven an improvement in PaO_2, median (range) +0.7 kPa (-0.4 to $+1.7$), $P < 0.05$, during spontaneous breathing by day. Bicarbonate ion concentration fell in seven patients -2.25 mmol/l (0 to -8.0), $P < 0.05$. At one year seven patients were still using the ventilator and $PaCO_2$ and bicarbonate ion concentration during the day had improved further compared to values at 6 months.

It is clear that NIPPV is less well tolerated and less effective in patients with COPD than in those with extrapulmonary restrictive disorders. Although there were significant numbers of dropouts from all the studies, three out of four did show that at least some patients with COPD could be ventilated

successfully at home using the nasal route. It is important to consider differences between these studies in view of the different outcomes and these are summarized in Table 9.1. Hypercapnia was a consistent feature in those patients who benefited from NIPPV. In studies using negative pressure devices, where benefit has been seen, it has usually been in those with daytime hypercapnia [24,26–28,40]. Secondly the duration of NIPPV may be important. The patients in the study of Strumpf *et al.* [38] only received NIPPV for 3 months, whereas in the others NIPPV continued for up to two years, and in one [39] arterial blood gas tensions were better at one year than after 6 months. The reason for this is not clear, but may relate to more complete acclimatization to the technique with time. Thirdly although all the patients in the series of Gay *et al.* [41], of Marino [37] and of Carroll and Branthwaite [31] started NIPPV as in-patients, those in the study of Strumpf *et al.* [38] were introduced to NIPPV as outpatients, albeit with considerable domiciliary support. Three of the four patients in the remaining study [39], who did not cope with the technique, were introduced to it as an outpatient. Success was greater when patients started NIPPV in hospital under close supervision. Finally, the choice of machine and mode of ventilation is important. Volume cycled ventilators were used in all studies except that of Strumpf, where the BiPAP was used. The BiPAP may not be sufficient to adequately control nocturnal hypoventilation in patients with a high impedance to inflation, because it is unable to generate inspiratory pressures greater than 22 cmH$_2$O [42]. Strumpf *et al.* used the timed mode because it is more likely to reduce inspiratory muscle effort than patient-initiated ventilation, but noted that approximately 25% of the night was spent with the patient breathing out of synchrony with the ventilator. Asynchrony between the patient and ventilator may cause marked

Table 9.1 Studies of nasal positive pressure ventilation in patients with COPD

	Carroll and Branthwaite [31]	Gay et al. [41]	Marino [37]	Strumpf et al. [38]	Elliott et al. [39]
Design	Uncontrolled	Uncontrolled	Uncontrolled	Crossover	Uncontrolled
Duration of NIPPV	18 months	10 months	Mean 20 months	3 months	One year
Acclimatization	Inpatient	Inpatient	Inpatient/acute	Outpatient	Outpatient $n = 4$ Inpatient $n = 8$
Ventilator type	Volume cycled	Volume cycled	Volume cycled	BiPAP	Volume cycled
Ventilator mode	Assist-control	Assist-control		Timed	Assist-control
Primary rationale for nocturnal NIPPV	To control nocturnal hypoventilation	To control nocturnal hypoventilation		To reduce respiratory muscle activity	To control nocturnal hypoventilation
Overnight monitoring of effectiveness of NIPPV	SaO_2 and continuous $TcCO_2$	SaO_2, continuous $EtCO_2$ and radial artery line	None	SaO_2 and spot $EtCO_2$	SaO_2 and continuous $TcCO_2$
Number completing study	3/4	3/4 (1 death – CVA)	4/9	7 of 19 enrolled	7 of 12 (1 death)
Daytime PaO_2 before and after NIPPV	Pre 6.0 (5.7–6.5) Post 7.1 (6.3–7.7) kPa, P = n.s.		Pre 8.4 ± 0.7 Post 8.7 ± 0.4 kPa, P = n.s.	Pre 8.0 ± 0.5 Post 8.3 ± 0.5 kPa, P = n.s.	Pre 6.8 (5.6–7) Post 6.6 (6.2–8.4) kPa, P = n.s.
Daytime $PaCO_2$ before and after NIPPV	Pre 8.2 (7.0–9.2) Post 7.1 (4.9–7.7) kPa, P < 0.02		Pre 8.1 ± 0.4 Post 5.9 ± 0.8 kPa, p < 0.03	Pre 6.3 ± 0.4 Post 6.7 ± 0.3 kPa, P = n.s.	Pre 7.9 (6.3–9.9) Post 6.6 (4.2–8.1) kPa, P < 0.05
Hypercapnia pre NIPPV	All	All	All	1/23	All

worsening of gas exchange with both negative [43] and positive pressure devices [44]. Carbon dioxide control during sleep was assessed on the basis of reduced spot measurements of end-tidal CO_2. This may have missed periods of hypoventilation, for instance associated with asynchrony, and in addition $EtCO_2$ is an unreliable measure of $PaCO_2$ in patients with severe airways obstruction.

In a preliminary report from the Royal Brompton Hospital [45] of long-term follow-up of 30 patients with COPD receiving NIPPV at home, the median duration of treatment was 2.2 years (range 0.08–5.92). Four patients died and the ventilator was withdrawn from five. The 5-year actuarial probability of continuing NIPPV of 43% (95% CI, 6–80%) was similar to that for survival in the oxygen-treated patients in the MRC long-term domiciliary oxygen study.

In conclusion, NIPPV can be used effectively in some patients with COPD. Experience with nPV has shown that, though feasible in small uncontrolled pilot studies, extension to a wider population has been disappointing. In the only controlled study there was no benefit from NIPPV [30]. Domiciliary oxygen therapy is of proven benefit in COPD [1,2], but although compliance was very good in the trials this is not always the case in routine clinical practice, the main reason being the restriction placed upon lifestyle by the need for 15 hours oxygen per day. Symptomatic patients, who gain subjective benefit from O_2 therapy, are more likely to comply with therapy, but asymptomatic patients tend to use oxygen for insufficient time to gain survival benefit [3,4]. The failure to control hypercapnia, which appears to be associated with a worse prognosis [1,46,47], is a further problem. These limitations suggest that NIPPV during sleep, which does not interfere with daytime activities and reduces CO_2 tension, may be better tolerated and improve survival in COPD. It is important to note that oxygen given only overnight was associated with a worse survival than that given continuously in the NOTT study of domiciliary oxygen [2]. However, quality of life is extremely important and better years rather than more years may be the patients' first requirement. The further place of NIPPV in the management of chronic ventilatory failure in COPD can only be determined by a large-scale randomized comparison with domiciliary oxygen therapy, and a multi-centre European trial is currently in progress.

Well-motivated hypercapnic patients are most likely to benefit from NIPPV and adequate education and acclimatization to the technique are essential. In-hospital initiation of ventilation is preferable, though more costly and the adequacy of control of nocturnal hypoventilation needs to be confirmed. Patients who are hypercapnic because of end-stage emphysema are unlikely to benefit because the elevated CO_2 is a consequence of an absence of functioning lung tissue, rather than due to secondary abnormalities of ventilatory drive and of the respiratory muscle pump.

Although it cannot currently be recommended as first-line treatment for hypercapnic patients with COPD, a trial of NIPPV should be considered in those cases deteriorating despite, or intolerant of, oxygen therapy. Muir [48] has suggested escalating treatment as the disease progresses, starting with oxygen given through mask or nasal cannulae and, if this is inadequate, transtracheally. If this fails, NIPPV is added and finally tracheostomy considered. Current suggestions for the use of NIPPV in COPD can be summarized as follows:

- Deterioration despite maximum conventional treatment or unable to tolerate oxygen therapy.
- Hypercapnia during spontaneous breathing by day.
- Not end-stage emphysema, i.e. moderately preserved transfer factor.

- Well-motivated.
- Inpatient acclimatization and education.
- Documented nocturnal hypoventilation breathing spontaneously.
- Documented control of nocturnal hypoventilation by NIPPV.

BRONCHIECTASIS

The pathophysiology of ventilatory failure in bronchiectasis is similar to that in COPD. Severe airways obstruction and hyperinflation occur in both conditions and worsening of blood gas tensions during sleep has been reported in patients with cystic fibrosis [49].

NIPPV has been used at home in four patients with cystic fibrosis and hypercapnic respiratory failure for up to 18 months [50]. All the patients had symptoms suggestive of overnight carbon dioxide retention confirmed by overnight monitoring and NIPPV was well tolerated. After a period of in-hospital treatment they were able to return home using the ventilator each night during sleep. This was associated with improved daytime arterial blood gas tensions, lessening of severe dyspnoea, subjective improvement in sleep and level of daily activities.

Similar results have been reported in older patients with bronchiectasis [51]. Of 16 patients starting NIPPV, one underwent heart/lung transplantation, two died and two were tracheostomized. The remainder were alive and well at up to 22 months after starting NIPPV, with improved quality of life and daytime blood gas tensions [51]. Hospital admissions each year were reduced from 1.5 per patient to 0.3 per patient. Leger *et al.* have reported an actuarial probability of continuing NIPPV at 5 years of 62% in 25 patients with bronchiectasis [52]. This compared favourably with sequelae of tuberculosis (60%), Duchenne muscular dystrophy (47%) and COPD (31%). A worse outcome in 12 patients with bronchiectasis, including cystic fibrosis was reported by Elliott *et al.* [45], with a median duration of NIPPV of 0.5 years (range 0.08 to 1.92), with seven patients dead and two transplanted. The differences in outcome reported in these studies may relate to patient selection and the time at which NIPPV was instituted.

MECHANISMS OF IMPROVEMENT IN DAYTIME FUNCTION IN COPD

The finding of improved arterial blood gas tensions during spontaneous breathing by day when ventilation has been assisted during sleep is perhaps surprising. It is helpful to consider the effects upon subsequent spontaneous ventilation in terms of changes in respiratory muscle function, the load upon it and the central drive to breathe (see Chapter 2). An improvement in blood gas tensions may occur if capacity or central drive increases or load is reduced (see Fig. 2.1).

Improved respiratory muscle function: one difficulty in exploring this hypothesis is the lack of any objective test of chronic fatigue. Some studies of non-invasive ventilation have cited increased respiratory muscle strength as evidence for the resolution of chronic fatigue [24–26,53]. However, tests of respiratory muscle strength require maximum voluntary efforts and an improvement in general well-being may have been responsible for the enhanced performance. In other studies improved arterial blood gas tensions, but without increased respiratory muscle strength, have been reported [41,54,55].

Secondly, although accessory muscle and diaphragmatic EMG activity can be reduced by both negative [56] and positive pressure devices [57], in most cases this has not been documented during the study. Rodenstein and colleagues [58] have show that accessory muscle and diaphragmatic EMG activity may not be reduced at all in naive patients and Ambrosino and colleagues [27], who measured integrated EMG activity during nPV, stated that activity was reduced by 50% only *temporarily*. The assumption that abolition of EMG activity occurring under ideal conditions, when ventilator controls have been adjusted to achieve this goal, also occurs during routine use may not be valid and it is therefore possible that the respiratory muscles were not rested at all in these studies. In some studies patients have been recruited during recovery from an acute exacerbation [26,40] and the changes seen may simply reflect the natural history of recovery, rather than any beneficial effect of assisted ventilation *per se*. Shapiro *et al.* [30] attempted to reduce respiratory muscle EMG activity using negative pressure devices in a randomized placebo controlled study. While this was not uniformly successful there was no evidence that respiratory muscle rest was of benefit. Further data are needed before the large scale application of respiratory muscle rest therapy is justified.

Restored chemosensitivity: improved chemosensitivity following the control of nocturnal hypoventilation has been shown in patients with OSA [59] and COPD [55]. Goldstein and co-workers [60] showed that non-invasive ventilation in patients with neuromuscular disease reduced the severity of nocturnal hypercapnia if ventilatory support was subsequently omitted, suggesting an increased central sensitivity to CO_2.

Reduced load: the effect of domiciliary ventilation upon respiratory system load in COPD has not been addressed in many studies. A small (non-significant) improvement in dynamic compliance and a correlation between the reduction in $PaCO_2$ during spontaneous breathing and a decrease in gas trapping (Spearman rank correlation coefficient (r_s) 0.85, $P < 0.05$) and in the residual volume (r_s 0.78, $P < 0.05$), suggesting reduced small airway obstruction and therefore a reduction in load, was seen in one study [55]. It was postulated that a reduction in lung water was one possible mechanism for these changes because if anything bronchodilator requirements were less following NIPPV. In most circumstances it is likely that any reduction in ventilatory load secondary to improved compliance is a relatively minor factor in the reversal of ventilatory failure.

Current evidence suggests that the pivotal action of NIPPV in reversing chronic ventilatory failure is its capacity to control nocturnal hypoventilation. It is quite possible that the efficiency of NIPPV, whether it provides all or only part of ventilation, whether the respiratory muscles are 'rested' or not, is of no great importance as long as nocturnal hypoventilation is controlled. Similarly, the particular technique of non-invasive ventilation may be largely irrelevant providing that the method used does control nocturnal hypoxaemia and hypercapnia.

The acceptance of any medical treatment depends upon the patient's perception of whether it is beneficial or not. Medical intervention that is unpleasant and is not perceived as beneficial will be poorly tolerated. There is no doubt that the results of NIPPV in patients with COPD are not as good as in those with chest wall deformity and stable neuromuscular disease. On top of this, NIPPV may be uncomfortable for the patient, particularly during acclimatization to the technique. Gastric distension and dry upper airway mucosae are particular problems. The balance towards benefit is therefore less and adequate motivation is an essential ingredient for a successful outcome. Patients may need considerable encouragement to persist during the early stages of NIPPV.

CONCLUSION

Non-invasive ventilation cannot be recommended as first line treatment for chronic ventilatory failure due to COPD, but it is a realistic alternative in selected patients when conventional therapy has failed.

The yearly cost of supplying and running a domiciliary nasal ventilator is about twice that of an oxygen concentrator. The patient will also require hospital admission to start NIPPV whereas this is not usually necessary when instituting LTOT. The social burden must also be calculated. Hypercapnic patients comprise a minority of those with COPD, and so it is likely that NIPPV would only ever be applicable in a small subgroup. While the suggestions given in this chapter for using NIPPV in COPD are appropriate in the light of current knowledge, it is clear that the results from trials comparing LTOT with LTOT/NIPPV which include quality of life measures should be the major determinant of the dissemination of this therapy in obstructive lung disease.

REFERENCES

1. Medical Research Council Working Party Report (1981) Long term domiciliary oxygen therapy in chronic hypoxic cor pulmonale complicating chronic bronchitis and emphysema. *Lancet*, **1**, 681–5.
2. Nocturnal Oxygen Therapy Trial Group (1980) Continuous or nocturnal oxygen therapy in hypoxaemic chronic obstructive lung disease, a clinical trial. *Ann. Intern. Med.*, **93**, 391–8.
3. Baudouin, S.V., Waterhouse, J.C., Tahtamouni, T. *et al.* (1990) Long term domiciliary oxygen treatment for chronic respiratory failure reviewed. *Thorax*, **45**, 195–8.
4. Walshaw, M.J., Lim, R., Evans, C.C. and Hind, C.R.K. (1990) Factors influencing compliance of patients using oxygen concentrators for long-term home oxygen therapy. *Respir. Med.*, **84**, 331–3.
5. Cooper, C.B., Waterhouse, J. and Howard, P. (1987) Twelve year clinical study of patients with hypoxic cor pulmonale given long term domiciliary oxygen therapy. *Thorax*, **42**, 105–10.
6. McNicholas, W.T. and Fitzgerald, M.X. (1984) Nocturnal deaths in patients with chronic bronchitis and emphysema. *Br. Med. J.*, **289**, 878.
7. Emery, C.J., Sloan, P.J., Mohammed, F.H. and Barer, G.R. (1977) The action of hypercapnia during hypoxia on pulmonary vessels. *Bull. Eur. Physiopathol. Respir.*, **13**, 763–76.
8. Arand, D.L., McGinty, D.J. and Littner, M.R. (1981) Respiratory patterns associated with hemoglobin desaturation during sleep in chronic obstructive pulmonary disease. *Chest*, **80**, 183–90.
9. Singh, B. (1984) Sleep apnea: a psychiatric perspective, in *Sleep and Breathing* (eds N.A. Saunders and C.E. Sullivan). Marcel Dekker, New York, pp. 403–22.
10. Calverley, P.M.A., Brezinova, V., Douglas, N.J. *et al.* (1982) The effect of oxygenation on sleep quality in chronic bronchitis and emphysema. *Am. Rev. Respir. Dis.*, **126**, 206–10.
11. Fleetham, J.A., West, P., Mezon, B. *et al.* (1982) Sleep, arousals, and oxygen desaturation in COPD. *Am. Rev. Respir. Dis.*, **126**, 429–33.
12. Berthon-Jones, M. and Sullivan, C.E. (1982) Ventilatory and arousal responses to hypoxia in sleeping humans. *Am. Rev. Respir. Dis.*, **125**, 632–9.
13. Hedemark, L. and Kronenberg, R. (1981) Ventilatory responses to hypoxia and CO_2 during natural and flurazepam induced sleep in normal adults. *Am. Rev. Respir Dis.*, **123**, 190 (Abstr.).
14. Guilleminault, C., Stoohs, R. and Duncan, S. (1991) Snoring (I). Daytime sleepiness in regular heavy snorers. *Chest*, **99**, 40–8.
15. Emmanuel, G.E., Smith, W.M. and Briscoe, W.A. (1966) The effect of intermittent positive pressure breathing and voluntary hyperventilation upon the distribution of ventilation and pulmonary blood flow to the lung in chronic obstructive lung disease. *J. Clin. Invest.*, **45**, 1221–3.
16. Fraimow, W., Cathcart, R.T. and Goodman, E. (1960) The use of intermittent positive pressure breathing in the prevention of carbon dioxide narcosis associated with oxygen therapy. *Am. Rev. Respir. Dis.*, **81**, 815–22.
17. Ayres, S.M., Kozam, R.L. and Lukas, D.S. (1963) The effects of intermittent positive pressure breathing on intrathoracic pressure, pulmonary mechanics and the work of breathing. *Am. Rev. Respir. Dis.*, **87**, 370–9.
18. Sukulmalchantra, Y., Park, S.S. and Williams, M.H. (1965) The effects of intermittent posi-

tive pressure breathing (IPPB) in acute venti-latory failure. *Am. Rev. Respir. Dis.*, **92**, 885–93.

19. Kamat, S.R., Dulfano, M.J. and Segal, M.S. (1962) The effects of intermittent positive pressure breathing (IPPB/I) with compressed air in patients with severe chronic nonspecific obstructive pulmonary disease. *Am. Rev. Respir. Dis.*, **86**, 360–80.

20. Curtis, J.K., Liska, A.P., Rasmussen, H.K. and Cree, E.M. (1968) IPPB therapy in chronic obstructive pulmonary disease. *J. Am. Med. Assoc.*, **206**, 1037–40.

21. Thornton, J.A., Darke, C.S. and Herbert, P. (1974) Intermittent positive pressure breathing (IPPB) in chronic respiratory disease. *Anaesthesia*, **29**, 44–9.

22. Emirgil, C., Sobol, B.J., Norman, J. *et al.* (1969) A study of the long-term effect of therapy in chronic obstructive pulmonary disease. *Am. J. Med.*, **47**, 367–77.

23. The Intermittent Positive Pressure Breathing Trial Group (1983) Intermittent positive pressure breathing therapy of chronic obstructive pulmonary disease. *Ann. Intern. Med.*, **99**, 612–20.

24. Gutierrez, M., Beroiza, T., Contreras, G. *et al.* (1988) Weekly cuirass ventilation improves blood gases and inspiratory muscle strength in patients with chronic airflow limitation and hypercarbia. *Am. Rev. Respir. Dis.*, **138**, 617–23.

25. Cropp, A. and Dimarco, A.F. (1987) Effects of intermittent negative pressure ventilation on respiratory muscle function in patients with severe chronic obstructive pulmonary disease. *Am. Rev. Respir. Dis.*, **135**, 1056–61.

26. Scano, G., Gigliotti, F., Duranti, R. *et al.* (1990) Changes in ventilatory muscle function with negative pressure ventilation in COPD. *Chest*, **97**, 322–7.

27. Ambrosino, N., Montagna, T., Nava, S. *et al.* (1990) Short term effect of intermittent negative pressure ventilation in COPD patients with respiratory failure. *Eur. Respir. J.*, **3**, 502–8.

28. Celli, B., Lee, H., Criner, G. *et al.* (1989) Controlled trial of external negative pressure ventilation in patients with severe chronic airflow limitation. *Am. Rev. Respir. Dis.*, **140**, 1251–6.

29. Zibrak, J.D., Hill, N.S., Federman, E.C. *et al.* (1988) Evaluation of intermittent long term

negative-pressure ventilation in patients with severe COPD. *Am. Rev. Respir. Dis.*, **138**, 1515–18.

30. Shapiro, S.H., Ernst, P., Gray-Donald, K. *et al.* (1992) Effect of negative pressure ventilation in severe chronic obstructive pulmonary disease. *Lancet*, **340**, 1425–9.

31. Carroll, N. and Branthwaite, M.A. (1988) Control of nocturnal hypoventilation by nasal intermittent positive pressure ventilation. *Thorax*, **43**, 349–53.

32. Ellis, E.R., Bye, P.T.B., Bruderer, J.W. and Sullivan, C.E. (1987) Treatment of respiratory failure during sleep in patients with neuro-muscular disease. *Am. Rev. Respir. Dis.*, **135**, 148–52.

33. Littner, N.R., McGinty, D.J. and Arand, D.L. (1980) Determinants of oxygen desaturation in the couse of ventilation during sleep in chronic obstructive pulmonary disease. *Am. Rev. Respir. Dis.*, **122**, 849–57.

34. Robert, D., Gerard, M., Leger, P. *et al.* (1983) Domiciliary ventilation by tracheostomy for chronic respiratory failure. *Rev. Fr. Mal. Resp.*, **11**, 923–36.

35. Stauffer, J.L., Olson, D.E. and Petty, T.L. (1981) Complications and consequences of endotracheal intubation and tracheostomy. *Am. J. Med.*, **70**, 65–75.

36. Muir, J.-F. and Cooperative Group (1987) Multicentre study of 259 severe COPD patients with tracheostomy and home mechanical ventilation, in Proceedings of the World Congress on Oxygen Therapy and Pulmonary Rehabilitation, Denver, 1987.

37. Marino, W. (1991) Intermittent volume cycled mechanical ventilation via nasal mask in patients with respiratory failure due to COPD. *Chest*, **99**, 681–4.

38. Strumpf, D.A., Millman, R.P., Carlisle, C.C. *et al.* (1991) Nocturnal positive-pressure ventilation via nasal mask in patients with severe chronic obstructive pulmonary disease. *Am. Rev. Respir. Dis.*, **144**, 1234–9.

39. Elliott, M.W., Simonds, A.K., Carroll, M.P. *et al.* (1992) Domiciliary nocturnal nasal intermittent positive pressure ventilation in hypercapnic respiratory failure due to chronic obstructive lung disease: effects on sleep and quality of life. *Thorax*, **47**, 342–8.

40. Corrado, A., Bruscoli, G., De Paola, E. *et al.* (1990) Respiratory muscle insufficiency in acute respiratory failure of subjects with severe COPD: treatment with intermittent negative pressure ventilation. *Eur. Respir. J.*, **3**, 644–8.

41. Gay, P.C., Patel, A.M., Viggiano, R.W. and Hubmayr, R.D. (1991) Nocturnal nasal ventilation for treatment of patients with hypercapnic respiratory failure. *Mayo Clin. Proc.*, **66**, 695–703.

42. Simonds, A.K. and Elliott, M.W. (1991) Use of the BIPAP ventilator for non-invasive ventilation: advantages and limitations. *Am. Rev. Respir. Dis.*, **143**(Suppl.), A585.

43. Simonds, A.K. and Branthwaite, M.A. (1985) Efficiency of negative pressure ventilatory equipment. *Thorax*, **40**, 213.

44. Rodenstein, D.O., Stanescu, D.C., Delguste, P. *et al.* (1989) Adaptation to intermittent positive pressure ventilation applied through the nose during day and night. *Eur. Respir. J.*, **2**, 473–8.

45. Elliott, M.W., Potter, N. and Simonds, A.K. (1993) Long-term follow-up of patients receiving domiciliary nasal intermittent positive pressure ventilation (NIPPV). *Eur. Respir. J.*, **6**, 381s (Abstr.).

46. Burrows, B. and Earle, R.H. (1969) Course and prognosis of chronic obstructive lung disease. *N. Engl. J. Med.*, **280**, 397–404.

47. Sahn, S.A., Nett, L.M. and Petty, T.L. (1980) Ten year follow-up of a comprehensive rehabilitation program for severe COPD. *Chest*, **77**(Suppl.), 311–14.

48. Muir, J.-F. (1992) Intermittent positive pressure ventilation (IPPV) in patients with chronic obstructive pulmonary disease (COPD). *Eur. Respir. Rev.*, **2**, 335–45.

49. Muller, N.L. Francis, P.W., Gurwitz, D. *et al.* (1980) Mechanism of hemoglobin desaturation during rapid-eye-movement sleep in normal subjects and patients with cystic fibrosis. *Am. Rev. Respir. Dis.*, **121**, 463–9.

50. Piper, A.J., Parker, S., Torzillo, P.J. *et al.* (1992) Nocturnal nasal IPPV stabilizes patients with cystic fibrosis and hypercapnic respiratory failure. *Chest*, **102**, 846–50.

51. Braghiroli, A. and Donner, C.F. (1992) Bronchiectasis. *Eur. Respir. Rev.*, **2**, 360–1.

52. Leger, P., Cornette, A., Bedicam, J.M. *et al.* (1993) Long term follow-up of severe chronic respiratory insufficiency patients (*n* = 276) treated by home nocturnal non invasive nasal IPPV (Abstract). 4th International Conference on Home Mechanical Ventilation, Lyons, France, 1993, p. 39.

53. Braun, N.M. and Marino, W.D. (1984) Effect of daily intermittent rest of respiratory muscles in patients with severe chronic airflow limitation (CAL). *Chest*, **85**, 59s–60s (Abstr.).

54. Mohr, C.H. and Hill, N.S. (1990) Long-term follow-up of nocturnal ventilatory assistance in patients with respiratory failure due to Duchenne-type muscular dystrophy. *Chest*, **97**, 91–6.

55. Elliott, M.W., Mulvey, D.A., Moxham, J. *et al.* (1991) Domiciliary nocturnal nasal intermittent positive pressure ventilation in COPD: mechanisms underlying changes in arterial blood gas tensions. *Eur. Respir. J.*, **4**, 1044–52.

56. Rochester, D.F., Braun, N.M. and Laine, S. (1977) Diaphragmatic energy expenditure in chronic respiratory failure. *Am. J. Med.*, **63**, 223–31.

57. Carrey, Z., Gottfried, S.B. and Levy, R.D. (1990) Ventilatory muscle support in respiratory failure with nasal positive pressure ventilation. *Chest*, **97**, 150–8.

58. Rodenstein D.O., Stanescu, D.C., Cuttita, G. *et al.* (1988) Ventilatory and diaphragmatic EMG responses to negative-pressure ventilation in airflow obstruction. *J. Appl. Physiol.*, **65**, 1621–6.

59. Berthon-Jones, M. and Sullivan, C.E. (1987) Time course of change in ventilatory response to CO_2 with long-term CPAP therapy for obstructive sleep apnea. *Am. Rev. Respir. Dis.*, **135**, 144–7.

60. Goldstein, R.S., Molotiu, N., Skrastins, R. *et al.* (1987) Reversal of sleep-induced hypoventilation and chronic respiratory failure by nocturnal negative pressure ventilation in patients with restrictive ventilatory impairment. *Am. Rev. Respir. Dis.*, **135**, 1049–55.

Nasal intermittent positive pressure ventilation as a 'bridge' to transplantation

MARK W. ELLIOTT

Heart/lung or lung transplantation has been generally available for the treatment of patients with end-stage, irreversible cardio-pulmonary disease for several years. As transplantation programmes have expanded so have the number of patients being considered for surgery. This coupled with a reduction in the number of donor organs available means that waiting times have become longer and in some patients respiratory failure worsens to the point where survival is compromised and ventilatory support becomes necessary. In this situation the choice lies between intubation and mechanical ventilation and non-invasive ventilation. There are little published data and no formal comparisons between the two techniques, but most experience of non-invasive ventilation in this clinical setting has been gained in patients with cystic fibrosis. Therefore 'bridging' to transplantation will be discussed primarily in this patient group. Although results can be extrapolated to other patients with obstructive lung disease (e.g. other causes of bronchiectasis and chronic obstructive airways disease), the same arguments do not apply in patients with end-stage fibrotic lung disease, in whom continuous positive airway pressure may be more appropriate.

Heart/lung transplantation has been performed successfully in patients with end-stage disease, with a 3-year survival approaching 70% [1]. Despite the success of the operation, a paucity of suitable donor organs is a major problem. Nasal intermittent positive pressure ventilation has been used successfully as a 'bridge' to transplantation [2,3] in patients who had deteriorated with severe hypoxaemia and hypercapnia to the point of requiring ventilatory assistance before donor organs became available. In the study of Hodson et al. [2] NIPPV was used in preference to intubation and mechanical ventilation in four patients with excellent results. There were no episodes of toxaemia or hypotension and patients were in a stable condition at the time of surgery. Duration of NIPPV ranged from three to 17 days. Two further patients, for whom suitable organs were not available, died 15 and 36 days after starting nasal ventilation, the latter from anastomotic problems and sepsis one week after bilateral single lung transplant, per-

Non-Invasive Respiratory Support. Edited by Anita Simonds. Published by Chapman & Hall, London. ISBN 0412 56840 3.

formed because a heart/lung block was not available. In contrast patients with cystic fibrosis intubated and ventilated conventionally have a high incidence of sepsis and subsequent death [4]. Many of these patients sustain damage to other vital organs rendering them unsuitable for heart/lung transplantation.

In patients successfully transplanted the duration of intubation (6–48 hours) and ICU stay following bridging using NIPPV was much shorter than following intubation and conventional ventilation [2]. In addition, patients trained in the technique pretransplant can use it more easily after surgery, which may enable them to avoid reintubation in the early postoperative period. Long-term outcome following transplantation appears no different from individuals who did not receive NIPPV preoperatively.

Ventilation via the nose is usually perceived as being less effective than when the patient is intubated, primarily because of inevitable leaks around the mask or through the mouth. However, comparison of the study of Hodson *et al.* [2] with that of Swami *et al.* [4] shows, surprisingly, that NIPPV is as effective as intubation and ventilation in improving arterial blood gas tensions. Nasal ventilation has the additional advantages that patients are able to cooperate with physiotherapy (see Chapter 14), can be involved in discussions about their management and can maintain nutrition and a degree of mobility. They can be managed on a general medical ward, rather than an Intensive Care Unit, which is more pleasant for the patients and their relatives and is considerably less expensive. Although additional humidification is not usually necessary for domiciliary nocturnal nasal ventilation because the nose continues to act as a natural humidifier, this is not true in patients with cystic fibrosis undergoing prolonged periods of assisted ventilation. The addition of a simple heat and moisture exchanger to the ventilator circuit may be sufficient, but formal humidification may be necessary to prevent excessive drying of secretions and mucosal surfaces (Fig. 10.1).

Because of the success of heart and heart/

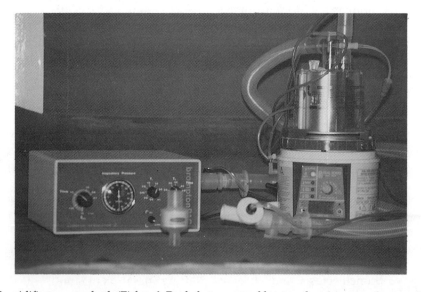

Fig. 10.1 Humidifiers: water bath (Fisher & Paykel at rear, and heat and moisture exchanger (Thermovent 1200, Portex Ltd) in foreground.

lung transplantation increasing numbers of patients have been considered for the operation and waiting lists have grown. Sadly many patients do not receive a transplant, although they can be kept alive for up to 29 months [5]. With such prolonged waits patients become increasingly ventilator-dependent, but most tolerate this well because nasal ventilation provides symptomatic relief of dyspnoea. However, pressure over the nasal bridge and skin breakdown may be a problem.

It is clear that patients can be kept alive for prolonged periods of time; however, the fact that currently many do not receive a transplant raises ethical questions about the use of nasal ventilation in end-stage cystic fibrosis. Although the outcome is disappointing, it is clearly better than that achieved following intubation and ventilation, and most of the patients successfully transplanted would certainly have died without ventilatory support. For those patients who do not receive a transplant, terminal care may be difficult, in that active treatment is continued aggressively in the hope that organs will become available. This puts a considerable strain on the patient and their family, but is a complication of waiting for a transplant rather than of nasal positive pressure ventilation *per se*.

The indications for starting NIPPV as a bridge to transplantation include intractable hypoxia despite increased inspired oxygen concentration, acidosis and, most commonly, increasing respiratory distress. The impedance to inflation is high and when volume-cycled machines are used patients are best ventilated with small tidal volumes and a rapid rate. Despite this, inflation pressures are usually high (approximately $40\,cmH_2O$), but there have been no reported cases of pneumothorax. Alternatively, pressure-cycled machines may be used. These may be particularly effective in patients in whom unloading of respiratory muscles, to alleviate respiratory distress, is the primary aim of nasal ventilation.

In conclusion, nasal intermittent positive pressure ventilation is the method of choice for patients with obstructive lung disease who need ventilatory support while awaiting transplantation. However, the problem of the paucity of suitable donor organs needs to be addressed if NIPPV is truly to be used as a means of prolonging life, rather than the act of dying.

REFERENCES

1. Yacoub, M.H., Banner, N.R., Khagani, A. *et al.* (1990) Heart–lung transplantation for cystic fibrosis and subsequent domino transplantation. *J. Heart Transplant.*, **9**, 459–67.
2. Hodson, M.E., Madden, B.P., Steven, M.H. *et al.* (1991) Non-invasive mechanical ventilation for cystic fibrosis patients – a potential bridge to transplantation. *Eur. Respir. J.*, **4**, 524–7.
3. Bellon, G., Mounier, M., Guidicelli, J. *et al.* (1992) Nasal intermittent positive pressure ventilation in cystic fibrosis. *Eur. Respir. Rev.*, **2**, 357–9.
4. Swami, A., Evans, T.W., Morgan, C.J. *et al.* (1991) Conventional ventilation as a bridge to heart–lung transplantation in cystic fibrosis. *Eur. Respir. J.*, **4**, 188s (Abstr.).
5. Le Bourgeois, M., Munck, A., Gerardin, M. *et al.* (1993) Nasal ventilation in children with cystic fibrosis (Abstract). 4th Internation Conference on Home Mechanical Ventilation, Lyons, France, 1993, p. 23.

11

Non-invasive ventilation in progressive neuromuscular disease and patients with multiple handicaps

ANITA K. SIMONDS

INTRODUCTION

The development of respiratory failure, often precipitated by aspiration pneumonia, is the common terminal event in most patients with progressive neuromuscular disorders. Motor neurone disease is the most prevalent of these disorders; other progressive conditions such as Duchenne muscular dystrophy and spinal muscular atrophy are considered in Chapter 12. It is clear that respiratory support may extend the life of these patients and alter the natural history of the condition, however the appropriateness of this intervention has not been systematically studied and so data are derived from several uncontrolled series. Groups with multiple handicaps in addition to respiratory failure comprise another category where the use of non-invasive ventilatory support is controversial. Quadriplegia and spina bifida are such conditions, and some information on prognostic factors and the use of NIPPV is available in these situations. Possible indications and contraindications to NIPPV in quadriplegia and spina bifida are presented.

MOTOR NEURONE DISEASE

There are approximately 5000 individuals with motor neurone disease (MND) in the UK. The incidence is 1 in 50 000 per year, with a mean age at onset of 56 years. The commonest presentation is with a constellation of upper and lower motor neurone signs in the spinal and bulbar territory (amyotrophic lateral sclerosis). Most texts suggest that respiratory symptoms in MND patients appear late and can be identified by simple spirometric monitoring. However, a presentation with over respiratory failure, or features of nocturnal hypoventilation, is well recognized [1]. Bulbar involvement is variable at the onset of the disease and is not related to prognosis; however bulbar symptoms are inevitable by the terminal phase. Median survival is around 2.5 years, but 25% of affected individuals may live for 5 years or more. Prognosis tends to be more favourable in younger patients.

The key respiratory issues in MND patients are dyspnoea, alveolar hypoventilation and ineffective cough related to respiratory

Non-Invasive Respiratory Support. Edited by Anita Simonds. Published by Chapman & Hall, London. ISBN 0412 56840 3.

muscle weakness, and aspiration and choking episodes secondary to bulbar involvement. Dyspnoea is unusual if vital capacity exceeds 50% predicted, but respiratory muscle function should be closely monitored if the VC falls below this value as respiratory decompensation commonly ensues within the next 12 months. Respiratory failure is virtually inevitable if VC falls below 30% predicted. Analysis of flow–volume loops will demonstrate abnormalities suggestive of upper airway dysfunction in many patients with MND. Not surprisingly, these findings occur more often, but not exclusively, in patients with bulbar involvement. Bulbar insufficiency worsens respiratory function by recurrent clinical and subclinical episodes of aspiration pneumonia. In addition to testing the gag reflex, swallowing ability can be usefully assessed at the bedside by watching the patient drink a glass of water rapidly. A more accurate evaluation of bulbar function can be obtained by video-fluoroscopy.

The development of respiratory failure early in the course of the disease denotes phrenic nerve involvement, often in conjunction with weakness of other respiratory muscles. It is this category of patients, particularly those with normal or only mildly impaired bulbar function and preserved limb strength, which respond best to non-invasive ventilation.

CHOICE OF VENTILATORY TECHNIQUE

Tracheostomy-IPPV (T-IPPV) has been used quite extensively in MND in the USA to circumvent progressive bulbar problems. In practice, selection of patients is often governed by the degree of insurance cover, extent of independent financial resources, and the availability of carers. Salamand *et al.* [2] report a 1-year survival of 24% in 24 MND patients receiving home T-IPPV. However, Oppenheimer and colleagues [3] have de-

monstrated an improved outcome, with up to 85% 1-year survival. In this series more than 50% of patients survived for 3 years or more using T-IPPV at home. A French group of patients using nasal–buccal ventilation or T-IPPV showed a transient improvement in pulmonary function, and it was possible to discharge all patients home [4].

Negative pressure techniques are unlikely to be helpful in MND as they may exacerbate upper airway dysfunction during sleep and worsen aspiration. nPV has been shown to reduce the symptoms of dyspnoea in several studies, however [5,6].

On theoretical grounds NIPPV should be helpful in patients with MND and early respiratory muscle involvement as it may help stabilize the upper airway during sleep [6]. We have seen excellent control of symptoms, increased confidence levels in the patient and family, and a relatively stable clinical state maintained for up to a year in patients with nocturnal hypoventilation started on NIPPV. Our practice is to treat symptomatic patients and keep asymptomatic individuals with hypoventilation under review. It is sometimes difficult to separate out nocturnal symptoms related to hypoventilation and those due to upper airway obstruction and aspiration. For this reason monitoring of respiration during sleep is mandatory before starting assisted ventilation. There is no evidence that NIPPV will reduce dyspnoea in patients who are normocapnic. Likewise, although continuous positive airway pressure (CPAP) might be predicted to help patients with nocturnal choking in the absence of hypoventilation, this can sometimes prove unhelpful and may only serve to burden the patient further.

TERMINAL CARE

In some units NIPPV is used as an intermediate phase before proceeding to T-IPPV once bulbar symptoms progress. This is less frequently seen in the UK as few centres carry out a tracheostomy in MND patients. Living wills may be an increasing feature in these patients. It is interesting to note that long-term ventilator assistance is elected in advance by only a small percentage of MND patients, but Oppenheimer [3] has pointed out that patient autonomy and decision-making is a sham unless patients are presented with adequate information and access to care options. All concerned should understand that if assisted ventilation is offered and accepted, patients should be able to opt to discontinue supportive therapy at any point. In practice it is easier to discontinue non-invasive methods than T-IPPV. In our experience it is more usual for the patient to want to continue with NIPPV in the terminal phase to maintain symptom relief. Increasing ventilator dependence is a certain accompaniment to this phase, and as weakness progresses many patients find the transition period from ventilatory support to self-ventilation inceasingly difficult. In this situation a deliberate reduction in the ventilator pressure of flow settings so that overnight CO_2 rises to betweem 6 and 7 kPa may help, without leading to a recurrence of symptoms of nocturnal hypoventilation. Anxiolytic medication, including morphine derivatives, and anticholinergic preparations to reduce secretions may also be of value. Advice on control of breathing and the forced expiration technique ('huffing') often helps. Each case should, however, be managed on an individual basis. The needs and feelings of carers should not be overlooked at this difficult time, and respite care made available. Some hospices are not familiar with the use of ventilators, and careful liaison regarding the uses and limitations of nasal ventilation with the patient's general practitioner and the hospice team is essential. The final event is still likely to be a chest infection. Use of opiates to relieve dyspnoea will allow the ventilator to be withdrawn without distress in the last days or hours of the patient's life.

QUADRIPLEGIA

As indicated previously (Chapter 7), patients with high cervical cord or bulbar lesions with no independent ventilatory capacity and an inability to clear secretions require tracheostomy-assisted ventilation. Expertise in managing these patients has been gained in many spinal injuries centres.

In recent years it has been demonstrated that some quadriplegic patients with minimal respiratory reserve may cope with long-term non-invasive methods, and where this is feasible, the option of non-invasive support should be pursued as it simplifies care and is preferable to patients [7]. Patients with unrecordable vital capacity may be able to self-ventilate for periods using glossopharyngeal ('frog') breathing.

The aetiology of quadriplegia ranges from traumatic cervical cord injury to stable neurological disorders (e.g. spina bifida, see below) to progressive neuromuscular disease. An individual with a cervical cord lesion rostral to C4 is likely to need ventilation immediately, those with a C4/5 injury may be able to support ventilation independently, but will decompensate in the presence of underlying chronic lung disease, spinal shock or the development of a chest infection. Critical to the well-being of these patients is physiotherapy and assisted coughing. Hyperinflation of the chest may be helpful in reducing the tendency to atelectasis and perhaps improving chest wall and pulmonary compliance, but there is little in the way of controlled trials in this area.

Assessment should include measurement of lung volumes, mouth pressures and overnight monitoring of respiration when symptoms of nocturnal hypoventilation are present, or vital capacity is less than 50% predicted. Sortor [7] has decribed the evaluation of the effectiveness of cough by separating it into several components:

1. The ability of the airway to respond to irritation.
2. Maximum inspiration: which is often reduced due to inspiratory muscle weakness.
3. Glottic closure: which is not usually a problem.
4. Contraction of the expiratory muscles against a closed area: often markedly impaired due to expiratory muscle weakness.
5. Opening of the airway: not usually a problem.

Assistance with coughing is required if the patient's inspiratory capacity is less than 50% predicted. This can be achieved by teaching the individual to stack spontaneous breaths, by using a hyperinflation device (e.g. Bird IPPB machine, Cape TC50) or increasing volume or flow settings during physiotherapy with the patient receiving NIPPV. The forced expiratory phase can be augmented by an abdominal thrust. Carers should be taught these techniques. A cough exsufflator (Emerson) has been developed which is widely used in some centres.

In a series of 62 quadriplegic patients treated at the Dallas Rehabilitation Institute from 1984 [7], 22 had a traumatic cervical cord lesion and 40 had neuromuscular disease (20 poliomyelitis, 9 muscular dystrophy, 6 spinal muscular atrophy, 3 motor neurone disease and 2 spina bifida). Of the cervical cord trauma group, 15 had lesions at C3 and above, 4 at C4 and 3 at C5. Nearly all were admitted with tracheostomies requiring ventilatory support, but it was possible to discharge 15 patients (68%) without a tracheostomy. Nine of these patients used nocturnal mask ventilation and five used negative pressure pneumojackets. Some used mouth ventilation or a pneumobelt as a ventilatory adjunct during the day. In the neuromuscular group, only 3 (7.5%) required a long-term

tracheostomy (2 with MND and one with muscular dystrophy). Of the remainder, 30 were supported with mask ventilation and 7 (including 5 children with spinal muscular atrophy) received negative pressure ventilation.

SPINA BIFIDA

Individuals with this condition require special consideration. As with patients with cervical cord injury, most spina bifida patients with lesions in the thoracic or lumbar region are wheelchair-bound, scoliotic and have impaired sphincter function. A proportion have hydrocepahalus, usually well-controlled by CSF shunt, and some are mentally handicapped. While the long-term outlook in those with lumbar/sacral defects may be good, death from respiratory failure is common in those with thoracic spinal defects.

Respiratory function in spina bifida patients may be compromised by mutiple factors including thoracic scoliosis, respiratory muscle weakness and central drive defects. In a series of spina bifida patients seen at the Royal Brompton Hospital ventilatory failure was associated with a thoracic spinal defect and vital capacity of less than 1000 ml [8]. Respiratory muscle strength and Cobb angle were not related to the degree of hypercapnia, but marked obesity was a potentially reversible factor in all patients with respiratory insufficiency. Sleep disordered breathing comprising a combination of hypoventilation and obstructive apnoea was seen in all patients and contributed to the progression of respiratory failure. It was corrected with nocturnal ventilatory support which reversed respiratory failure effectively [9] (Fig. 11.1). Despite the level of physical handicap, the quality of life in spina bifida patients receiving domiciliary NIPPV was no different from other groups, including those with idiopathic scoliosis and previous poliomyelitis [9]. However, quality of life measures are not

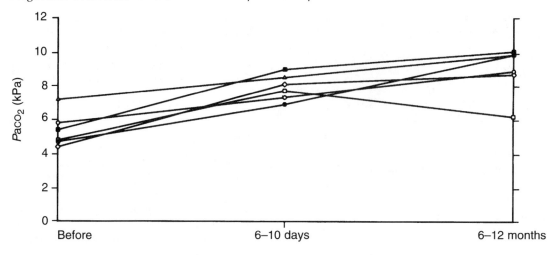

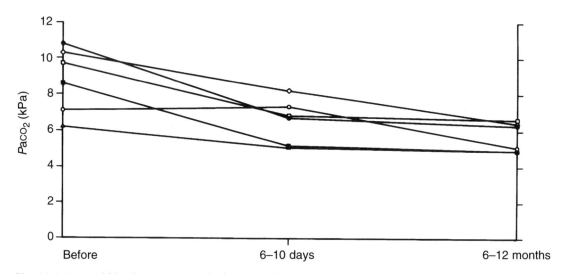

Fig. 11.1 Arterial blood gas tensions before and after NIPPV in spina bifida patients.

available before and after the institution of assisted ventilation.

CONCLUSIONS

Non-invasive ventilatory support is feasible in patients with progressive neuromuscular disease and may facilitate discharge from hospital and simplify care in quadriplegic individuals. The central issues are relief of symptoms, quality of life and patient automony. Medical attendants also have a duty to use these techniques cost-effectively. There is little controlled data in this area and further work on quality of life in both patients and carers, and long-term outcome, is required. In the meantime a wider scientific and public debate on the ethical aspects of respiratory support in these conditions should be encouraged.

REFERENCES

1. Al-Shaikh, B., Kinnear, W., Higenbottam, T.W. *et al.* (1986) Motor neurone disease presenting as respiratory failure. *Br. Med. J.*, **292**, 1325–6.
2. Salamand, J., Robert, D., Leger, P. *et al.* (1991) Definitive mechanical ventilation via tracheostomy in end-stage amyotrophic lateral sclerosis (Abstract). 3rd International Conference on Pulmonary Rehabilitation and Home Ventilation, Denver, 1991, p. 50.
3. Oppenheimer, E.A. (1992) Amyotrophic lateral sclerosis. *Eur. Respir. Rev.*, **2**, 323–9.
4. Goulon, M. and Goulon-Goeau, C. (1989) Sclerose lateral amyotrophique et assistance respiratoire. *Rev. Neurol.*, **145**, 293–8.
5. Sawicka, E.H., Loh, L. and Branthwaite, M.A. (1988) Domiciliary ventilatory support; an analysis of outcome. *Thorax*, **43**, 31–5.
6. Howard, R.S., Wiles, C.M. and Loh, L. (1989) Respiratory complications and their management in motor neuron disease. *Brain*, **112**, 1155–70.
7. Sortor, S. (1991) Pulmonary issues in quadriplegia. *Eur Respir. Rev.*, **2**, 330–4.
8. Varnava, A., Woodhead, M., Steven, M.H. and Simonds, A.K. (1991) Respiratory failure in spina bifida: aetiology and prognostic features. *Am. Rev. Respir. Dis.*, **145**, A863.
9. Dilworth, J.P., Potter, N. and Simonds, A.K. (1994) Outcome of nasal ventilation in spina bifida patients with hypercapnic respiratory failure. *Eur. Respir. J.*, **7**, 415s.

12

Paediatric non-invasive ventilation

ANITA K. SIMONDS

INTRODUCTION

The number of children receiving assisted ventilation at home is increasing. A recent USA survey of domiciliary ventilation [1] showed that the largest subgroup of recipients is comprised of children under the age of 11 years and this category and shown the most rapid growth over the past 5 years. In 1992 22% (47/216) of ventilator-assisted individuals in the state of Minnesota were in the paediatric age range. Robinson [2] has examined the care of long-term ventilator-dependent children in the UK. Twenty-four children were identified, but this study focused on children receiving ventilation by day and night (usually due to cervical cord trauma, neuromuscular or parenchymal lung disease), and excluded a far larger group of individuals treated with non-invasive methods predominantly at night. The main underlying diagnosis in this latter group is neuromuscular disease.

Patients with parenchymal lung disease such as bronchopulomary dysplasia are likely to require tracheostomy-IPPV (T-IPPV), as are those with high cervical lesions who need 24-hour ventilatory support. Non-invasive methods of ventilation are suitable in other subgroups, especially for nightime support, and there is a growing body of experience in this area. In some situations T-IPPV is preferable because of the age of the child, in other instances T-IPPV was previously the standard treatment and has been superseded by nasal ventilation. Where available, outcome data and the practical problems associated with these indications will be compared. Most information exists on domiciliary ventilation in childhood spinal muscular atrophy, Duchenne muscular dystrophy, congenital myopathies and chest wall disease, and so these areas will be covered in detail. To set ventilatory activity in neuromuscular disease in perspective, the European Alliance of Muscular Dystrophy Associations estimates that the prevalence of spinal muscular atrophy (types 1 and 2), Duchenne muscular dystrophy and congenital myopathies in Europe is approximately 6000, 18000 and 15000 cases, respectively.

SPINAL MUSCULAR ATROPHY

This anterior horn cell disease is inherited as an autosomal recessive trait. Chromosome mapping has shown that the defective gene is located on the long arm of chromosome 5 [3]. On developmental grounds spinal muscular atrophy (SMA) can be classified into types I–III, as illustrated in Table 12.1.

Individuals with all forms of SMA are at risk from nocturnal hypoventilation and ultimately diurnal respiratory failure. While

Non-Invasive Respiratory Support. Edited by Anita Simonds. Published by Chapman & Hall, London. ISBN 0412 56840 3.

Table 12.1 Classification of spinal muscular atrophy

	Clinical features	*Inheritance*
Type I Werdnig–Hoffman disease	Hypotonic at birth. Unable to hold head up. 　May be accompanying brain stem 　abnormality and pulmonary aplasia Death before the age of 4 years in 95%	Autosomal recessive
Type I Inter–mediate	Able to hold head up, unable to sit Usually diagnosed in first year Often recurrent respiratory tract infections	Autosomal recessive
Type II Kugelberg–Welander	Able to sit up, unable to walk Proximal and intercostal muscle involvement. 　Diaphragm often spared. Scoliosis	Autosomal recessive. Less common dominant and X-linked forms
Type III	Symmetrical proximal weakness. Scoliosis Respiratory insufficiency in young adulthood	

patients with type I SMA may require ventilation within several months of birth, those in the type I intermediate group and type II often require ventilatory support in the first two years of life and individuals with type III SMA develop respiratory insufficiency in the second, third or fourth decades, depending on the extent of respiratory muscle involvement and the severity of scoliosis. Extensive experience in providing ventilatory support for SMA children has been reported by Barois and colleagues [4]. Clearly the logistical problems are most complex in providing ventilatory assistance to children with Type I SMA. However, Barois has demonstrated favourable results in 22 children with Wernig–Hoffmann disease discharged home using T-IPPV. This team advocate the use of home nasal ventilation where more than 4 hours a day ventilatory assistance is required, in the absence of swallowing problems and/or marked bronchial secretions. Fourteen children with SMA over the age of 2 years have been treated with NIPPV (mean age 10 years) and nine children under the age of 2 years (mean age 15.5 months). A tracheostomy was subsequently performed in a minority of patients.

Good quality of life may be maintained into adolescence and beyond in Type I intermediate and Type II forms, although insufficient time has elapsed to judge long-term results with NIPPV. Mental handicap is not a feature of SMA and many children are able to participate in normal schooling. In addition to symptom control and normalization of arterial blood gas tensions, positive pressure ventilation may be particularly helpful in fostering the normal development of alveoli and the chest wall, as indicated by a progressive fall in vital capacity/total lung capacity ratio in untreated SMA type II patients and stable/increasing lung volumes in cases receiving assisted ventilation [4]. Severe chest wall recession is a characteristic feature of SMA as shown in a child with type I intermediate disease in Fig. 12.1. It is possible that these deformities may be modified by adequate ventilation. Careful attention also needs to be paid to the development of scoliosis and contractures which compromise respiration and limit mobility.

103

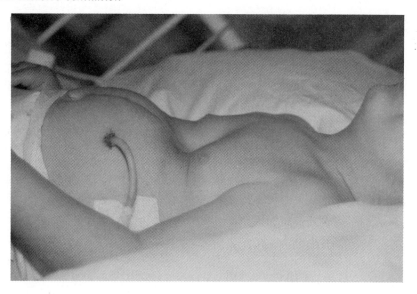

Fig. 12.1 Chest wall deformity in spinal muscular atrophy. This child also has a feeding gastrostomy.

DUCHENNE MUSCULAR DYSTROPHY

This most common muscular dystrophy in childhood is inherited as an X-linked recessive disorder with an incidence of around 1 in 3500 live male births. The gene responsible for DMD and its milder variant Becker muscular dystrophy has been identified and its gene product (dystrophin) characterized. Lack of dystrophin appears to lead to the most severe forms of Duchenne muscular dystrophy (DMD), probably by causing muscle membrane dysfunction, fibrotic and fatty change and ultimately muscle atrophy.

In affected boys motor delay is usually noticed by the age of 2 or 3 years. In a French series, Rideau *et al.* [5] showed that on average patients become wheelchair-bound by the age of 10 years and 50% develop a significant scoliosis. Without ventilatory support the mean age at death is around 19 years, with 73% of deaths occurring as a consequence of hypercapnic respiratory failure. Just under 20% of patients died during an acute infective exacerbation and 9% of deaths were attributed to cardiac disease.

The evolution of lung function changes in DMD has been divided into three strages: an initial phase during the first 10 years where forced vital capacity (FVC) increases as predicted; a second phase during which lung volumes plateau as muscle weakness +/− socliosis becomes manifest; and a final phase in which FVC initially falls slowly, but may decline by as much as 250 ml/year in the last few years of life [6]. Peak vital capacity is a prognostic factor, as Rideau *et al.* [5] showed that a peak VC of less than 1200 ml was associated with an average age at death of 15.3 years, while values in excess of 1700 ml resulted in survival to 21 years. Cardiac involvement takes the form of conduction defects and a dilated or hypertrophic cardiomyopathy. Dilated cardiomyopathy as evidenced by cardiomegaly and left ventricular dysfunction is the commonest abnormality. Nigro *et al.* [7] found preclinical evidence of cardiac disease in 25% of DMD patients under the age of 6 years and 59% between the ages of 6 and 10 years. Clinically apparent cardiac involvement was present in all patients by the age of 18 years, and about 72% of these patients were symptomatic. This is important as breathlessness and fatigue due to cardiac failure may be erroneously attributed to respiratory insufficiency.

The first signs of respiratory compromise occur during sleep. REM sleep-related hypoventilation is common when vital capacity is less than 30% predicted and increases with age [8].

Obstructive apnoeas occur in a proportion of patients and may predate the development of hypoventilation [9]. A Cheyne–Stokes pattern of breathing may been seen in DMD patients with severe cardiomyopathy. Patients with mild to moderate nocturnal hypoxaemia often remain asymptomatic. Most authorities recommend that routine sleep studies are not indicated, but monitoring should be carried out in the presence of symptoms of nocturnal hypoventilation [9].

Long-term ventilatory assistance in DMD remains a controversial issue despite the fact that various forms of ventilatory assistance have been employed in DMD patients for at least 20–30 years [5,10]. Concerns focus on the fact that DMD may progress rapidly with reduction in peripheral muscle strength accompanying respiratory muscle involvement so that as a consequence the individual may end up ventilator-dependent and immobile, with an unacceptable quality of life.

Before the mid-1980s the options available for ventilatory support were T-IPPV, mouthpiece ventilation, negative pressure devices, the pneumobelt and rocking bed. Alexander *et al.* [10] report a series of patients with late stage DMD who received ventilatory assistance for up to 7 years. Patients used a variety of techniques including mouthpiece-IPPV, cuirass, pneumowrap and rocking bed, with the aim of continuing non-invasive methods long term and avoiding tracheostomy. Treatment was begun in response to symptomatic hypercapnia and ventilatory support was continued for an average of 3.4 years. Care was delivered in the community and patients were reported to have a meaningful quality of life. By contrast, Rideau and co-workers [5] used IPPV via a fenestrated tracheostomy in a series of DMD patients following the development of acute-on-chronic respiratory failure or symptoms of nocturnal hypoventilation. All subjects had a moderate to severe scoliosis and vital capacity of less than 550 ml. A tracheostomy was performed between the ages of 16 and 23 years and none of the patients required daytime ventilatory support, allowing them to complete schooling and carry on with other activities. It is notable that several patients died of complications related to the tracheostomy.

Hill [11] examined the effects of negative pressure in DMD patients aged around 23 years with an average vital capacity of approximately 300 ml. Monitoring of respiration during sleep confirmed that nearly all patients experienced more than five episodes per hour of sleep disordered breathing accompanied by sleep disruption and desaturation during negative pressure ventilation. These episodes were predominantly obstructive apnoeas or hypopnoeas. Supplemental oxygen was not helpful in alleviating respiratory disturbances, and tended to prolong the duration of events. The authors found it necessary to use nasal CPAP in two patients and a tracheostomy in another as an adjunct to nPV. This combination adds considerably to the complexity of treatment.

Mouth piece-intermittent positive pressure ventilation (MIPPV) has also been employed effectively in DMD [12], and may be used in addition to other modes as a ventilatory adjunct during the day.

Several groups have demonstrated desaturation precipitated by upper airway obstruction in patients using nPV and have shown that a switch to NIPPV can eliminate the problem [13,14]. Recurrent aspiration during nPV may be a particular problem in individuals with reduced bulbar reflexes [6]. For these reasons NIPPV is probably the treatment of choice in DMD, although a preliminary study comparing different ventilatory modes in DMD produced inconclusive results [15].

There has been no controlled study of the use of assisted ventilation in DMD patients with nocturnal and diurnal hypercapnia. However, the long term effects of NIPPV have been explored by comparing the clinical course and pulmonary function in five hypercapnic patients who recieved NIPPV and a control group of five patients who did not receive ventilatory support [16]. Over a 2-year period all the subjects receiving NIPPV survived, whereas four out of five of the control subjects died (mean survival 9.7 months). After 6 months, mean loss of vital capacity and maximal voluntary ventilation was significantly greater in the control group. Although these subjects were not randomized to treatment and there was a trend to older age, higher $PaCO_2$ and smaller tidal volumes in the control group, these results strongly suggest NIPPV is of value in prolonging survival in DMD patients. Hill [17] has concluded that the evidence for nocturnal NIPPV in symptomatic, hypercapnic patients with DMD is now so persuasive that research activity should be focused on *how* it works, rather than *whether* it works.

A caveat is that quality of life has not been comprehensively investigated in DMD patients receiving home ventilation, or their carers – which is a major omission. It should also be remembered that nocturnal ventilation is just one component of the management of these patients. Advice regarding physiotherapy, sputum clearance, nutrition, assessment of scoliosis and aids to daily living all form essential parts of a comprehensive care plan [18].

PROPHYLACTIC USE OF NON-INVASIVE VENTILATION IN DMD

The above reports describe the use of assisted ventilation in individuals with established, *symptomatic* chronic hypoventilation. As an extension of this work it has been suggested that the employment of non-invasive ventilation earlier in the course of the disease before the development of overt symptoms may have an even more beneficial effect on the natural history of the condition, by reducing the decline in lung function. A French study [19] has addressed this issue and shown *no* evidence that the early introduction of non-invasive ventilation in normocapnic DMD patients improves lung function or offers a survival advantage, and indeed harm may result if ventilation is not adequately monitored. Not surprisingly, the treatment was poorly tolerated. *Prophylactic* use of non-invasive ventilation in DMD therefore *cannot* be recommended [20].

NON-PROGRESSIVE/SLOWLY PROGRESSIVE MUSCLE DISORDERS

LIMB GIRDLE MUSCULAR DYSTROPHY

Generalizations are inadvisable in this condition, as problems with diagnosis have led to cases of Becker muscular dystrophy, spinal muscular atrophy and congenital muscular dystrophy being misclassified as limb girdle muscular dystrophy (LGMD) in the past. The course of the disease can also be variable. Although many patients remain ambulant until adulthood, a rapidly progressive form of the LGMD mimicking Duchenne muscular dystrophy can occur in childhood. LGMD is inherited as an autosomal recessive disorder and overall progression in members of an affected family usually follows a similar pattern, with onset of respiratory failure at roughly the same age. Disproportionate early involvement of the respiratory muscles appears relatively common, so that some individuals remain ambulant but dependent on nocturnal hypoventilation. Cardiac complications are rare [21].

CONGENITAL MUSCULAR DYSTROPHY

The diagnostic category of congenital muscular dystrophy (CMD) is used to define a group of patients with weakness with or without hypotonia at birth, in whom a muscle biopsy shows features compatible with a dystrophic process [21]. The degree of weakness is highly variable, but respiratory and facial muscles can be involved, and contractures plus scoliosis are consistent features (Fig. 12.2). Although generalized weakness may be static, respiratory decompensation can occur during childhood or adolescence due to a progressive socliosis and fall in respiratory muscle strength. In a series of CMD children treated by Barois *et al.* [22],

one-third had sufficient limb strength to continue walking, but diaphragm weakness was common. NIPPV was used in the majority of cases aged 2–10 years; a few patients required tracheostomy. In seven patients with CMD seen at the Royal Brompton/ Hammersmith Hospital, respiratory failure occurred between the ages of 4 and 15 years. Symptoms and arterial blood gas tensions were controlled using nocturnal ventilatory support, allowing the individuals to continue normal schooling during the day.

MYOPATHIES

The congenital myopathies comprise the following conditions.

- Central core disease.
- Minicore disease.
- Nemaline myopathy.
- Congenital fibre type disproportion.

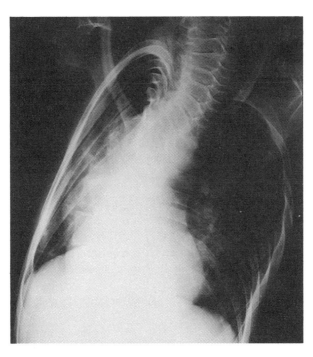

Fig. 12.2 Chest radiograph of an 11-year-old child with congenital scoliosis who developed respiratory failure in association with a rapidly progressive scoliosis.

- Mitochondrial myopathy.
- Minimal change myopathy.

Respiratory muscle weakness appears to be particularly associated with nemaline and mitochondrial myopathies.

Of the metabolic myopathies, Pompe's disease (acid maltase deficiency) can produce classic features of diaphragm weakness as the most early manifestation of the disease. A severe form in childhood may resemble SMA.

CENTRAL HYPOVENTILATION DISORDERS

Congenital hypoventilation is rare. In affected individuals the metabolic control of ventilation is abnormal, but behavioural control is retained. Infants usually present in the first few days of life with apnoeic episodes and cyanosis. Acquired central hypoventilation can occur as a consequence of encephalitis, following trauma or due to brain stem lesions. A further group may develop hypoventilation as a result of hypothalamic/pituitary disease. In a Royal Brompton series of these patients the sensation of dyspnoea and hypercapnic ventilatory drive were absent and the onset of respiratory failure was in late childhood or adolescence. Obesity, anterior and posterior pituitary deficiency and, in some cases, aberrant temperature and pain sensation may complicate the picture. Whereas ventilation remains adequate during the day, profound hypoventilation occurs during sleep, so these individuals can derive benefit from nocturnal non-invasive ventilation. In one patient a progressive deterioration in respiratory control during the day was seen after 7 years of nocturnal ventilation.

CHEST WALL DISORDERS

EARLY ONSET SCOLIOSIS

Although congenital and juvenile scoliosis are a risk factor for the development of res-

piratory insufficiency (Chapter 2), overt respiratory failure in these patients is unusual in childhood unless other problems such as muscle weakness, rigid spine syndrome or parenchymal lung disease are present (Fig. 12.3). Scoliosis can also complicate inherited syndromes such as Marfan's syndrome, neurofibromatosis amd Ehlers–Danlos syndrome, but there are few data on respiratory decompensation in the paediatric age group in these disorders.

RIGID SPINE SYNDROME

The rigid spine syndrome is an interesting but poorly defined clinical entity characterized by stiffness and marked reduction in flexion of the dorsolumbar and cervical spine. The term was coined by Dubowitz [21]. It is plain that the features of the rigid spine syndrome accompany conditions such as congenital muscular dystropy, the Emery–Dreifuss syndrome and minimal change myopathy, but at present it seems sensible to keep these as separate diagnostic labels until further genetic studies establish the molecular basis of the disorders. The evidence available would suggest that an underlying myopathy is present as spinal electromyogram shows a myopathic pattern and creatinine phosphokinase (CPK) level is often elevated. Spinal rigidity seems to have a marked effect on the mechanical efficiency of the respiratory and accessory muscles, in addition to reducing chest wall compliance. It is possible that cervical spine immobility predisposes the individual to upper airway obstruction. This combination of factors means that respiratory failure can develop insidiously in the presence of a straight spine and relatively well-preserved vital capacity (e.g. >1.5 litres).

In a group of nine patients with rigid spine syndrome (aged 13–32 years) [23], four patients who developed respiratory failure had a mean vital capacity of 40% predicted

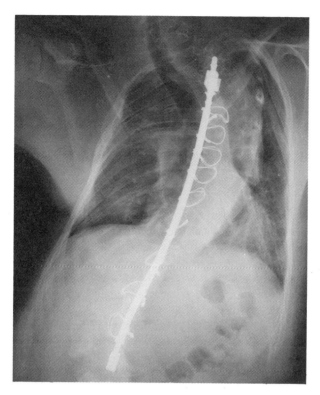

Fig. 12.3 Chest radiograph of a 14-year-old patient with congenital scoliosis, tracheo-oesophageal fistula and left lower lobe brochiectasis who developed respiratory failure at the age of 10 years.

compared to a mean value of 68% predicted in individuals who remained normocapnic. A fatal cardiomyopathy has been reported in one patient with the rigid spine syndrome [24]. Cardiac arrhythmias are a feature of the Emery–Dreifuss syndrome.

PRACTICAL POINTS

DIAGNOSTIC UNCERTAINTY

A firm diagnosis is essential to provide prognostic information, plan future care and facilitate genetic counselling of the family. Advances in the interpretation of muscle biopsy histology have improved the diagnosis of many childhood neuromuscular conditions, but diagnostic uncertainty can be a problem when a child presents acutely in

respiratory failure. It is advisable to make every attempt to secure an unequivocal diagnosis in each case so that outcome can be properly assessed.

IDENTIFICATION OF HIGH RISK CASES AND MONITORING

Regular follow-up of children with a vital capacity of less than 50% predicted is recommended. In DMD patients a decline in lung function is often seen within several years of the loss of ambulation. Symptoms of nocturnal hypoventilation such as headaches, poor sleep and fatigue are well known, but in young children irritablilty, poor concentration and failure to thrive may be more prominent. In wheelchair-bound patients cyanosis is frequently first observed when the child is eating or getting dressed. These features are an indication for nocturnal monitoring of respiration by oximetry and, where possible, measurement of transcutaneous/ end-tidal CO_2, oronasal airflow and chest wall movement to establish the contribution of central hypoventilation and upper airway obstruction. Our practice in paediatric cases is to use nocturnal oximetry with transcutaneous CO_2 monitoring (Hewlett Packard model 47210A or Radiometer TINA system), and the Densa Pneumograph 600 to differentiate between obstructive and central respiratory disturbances (Fig. 12.4). Both the Radiometer transcutaneous system and Densa Pneumograph can be applied in the home with relative ease, and have the advantage of being suitable for monitoring patients of all sizes, from a neonate to 130 kg adult! Screening pulse oximetry is employed in some centres. If the child has slept well, a normal SaO_2 trace probably excludes significant sleep disordered breathing. Traces may be equivocal, however, in which case more detailed studies (as above) are indicated.

Considerable experience is required in the interpretation of the results.

An additional indication for noctural respiratory support is recurrent respiratory infections associated with ventilatory insufficiency. For example, mask ventilation has been used in a 19-month-old child with intermediate SMA (Fig. 12.5) who had been hospitalized elsewhere for 6 months with recurrent right middle and lower lobe pneumonia (Fig. 12.6), hypoxaemia and nocturnal hypercapnia. The introduction of nocturnal bi-level pressure support delivered by a full facemask, facilitated discharge home and no further hospital admissions have been required during 12 months of follow-up. We have also used nocturnal CPAP via full facemask in a 3-year-old with SMA who presented with recurrent chest infections necessitating intubation and conventional ventilation on two occasions in the previous 3 months. In this child diurnal and nocturnal $PaCO_2$ were normal and so CPAP was used in preference to NIPPV. In 18 months of follow-up there have been no further chest infec-

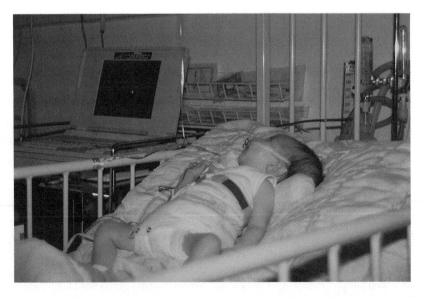

Fig. 12.4 Paediatric monitoring of respiration during sleep using Densa Pneumograph 600 system.

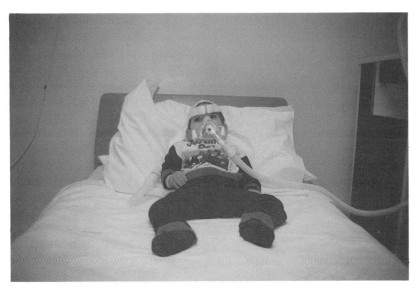

Fig. 12.5 A 19-month-old infant with intermediate spinal muscular atrophy receiving facemask ventilation using the BiPAP ventilator.

tions, ABG tensions remain stable and growth velocity has markedly increased.

CHOICE AND INTRODUCTION OF VENTILATORY SYSTEM

Tracheostomy-IPPV will be needed for patients with either inadequate bulbar reflexes or extreme ventilator dependence. Previously it has been advocated that negative pressure ventilation is advisable in children under the age of 6 years who require nocturnal ventilatory support, and these techniques are used extensively in some centres. However, Barois [4] has cautioned that nPV in early childhood can create chest wall deformity, and it is now clear that nasal or facemask delivery of IPPV can be employed in children of less than 2 years (Fig. 12.5). Consequently, it is no longer sensible to offer firm guidelines on the basis of age. As indicated above, CPAP may be suitable for children with recurrent chest infections and nocturnal hypoxaemia in the absence of marked CO_2 retention.

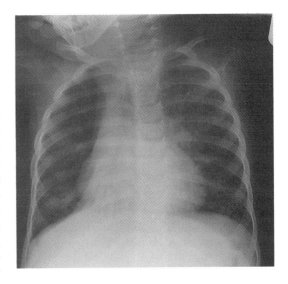

Fig. 12.6 Chest radiograph of the child in Fig. 12.5 who presented with recurrent right middle lobe and lower lobe pneumonia.

111

Masks

In very small children it may be necessary to use customized nasal or full facemasks, although commercially available masks are now produced in petite and paediatric sizes (Respironics Inc., Rescare Ltd). Rescare Ltd have developed a nasal mask and headgear suitable for neonatal application in cases of central sleep apnoea (Fig. 3.13). The smallest size Adam circuit nasal pillows (to date) accommodate children of around 10 years of age or above.

Ventilator

In the French series of paediatric cases [4] volume-preset ventilators were used (Eole 1A/E, 2A/E, Monnal D, Lifecare PLV-100). In 30 Royal Brompton/Hammersmith children started on NIPPV over half use the BiPAP S/T ventilator (Respironics Inc.) and most of the remainder use the Nippy (Thomas Respiratory Systems) or OP90 (Taema). In obese teenagers with Duchenne muscular dystrophy occasionally a more powerful volume-preset ventilator, e.g. BromptonPAC (Pneupac Ltd) has been required to achieve satisfactory control of ABG tensions. Below the age of 18 months triggering of the BiPAP can be unreliable – we have found the PLV-100 (Lifecare) effective in this situation.

STARTING NIPPV

Acclimatization to the ventilatory system is a highly individual affair and needs to be titrated to the child. If NIPPV is being started electively this is best achieved by an admission to hospital for a few days. Involvement of the parents or carer from the start of treatment is essential to build confidence and reduce anxiety. Young children and those with weakness of the small muscles of the hands or shoulder girdle will need help in securing the mask. Carers should be advised not to pull the straps securing the mask too

tight as this distorts the contours of the mask and may lead to a nasal sore. Fortunately nasal bridge lesions seem less common in children. In those of around 8 years of age or more, who are able to understand the rationale for treatment, NIPPV can be introduced at the child's pace during the day. Not surprisingly, boredom is a great enemy during intensive NIPPV use and can be alleviated using videos, story telling and games adapted to the situation. Encouragement and gentle persistence is necessary in the early stages. For younger children the chances of success are increased by introducing the mask at night after the child has dozed off. Full face masks are often helpful, but inveterate thumbsuckers may be adequately ventilated with a nasal mask. The selection of masks is discussed in Chapter 3. Oximetry and transcutaneous CO_2 monitoring can be employed to establish appropriate ventilator settings, supplemented by arterialized ear lobe blood gas sampling which is well tolerated by children. We perform overnight monitoring of oximetry and transcutaneous CO_2 to ensure control of nocturnal hypoventilation before discharge home (Fig. 12.7). If ventilation is required during the day in a child using a wheelchair, mask or mouthpiece ventilation can be continued using batter powered equipment (e.g. Lifecare PLV-100). Alternatively a pneumobelt can be used.

DISCHARGE HOME

The home care of a ventilator-dependent child poses particular problems, which are magnified if the condition is progressive. Although the child is more likely to thrive in the home environment, the family can experience high levels of stress [25,26] so that psychosocial support for caregivers is essential. Financial problems often add to the burden. Discharge planning is discussed in Chapter 14.

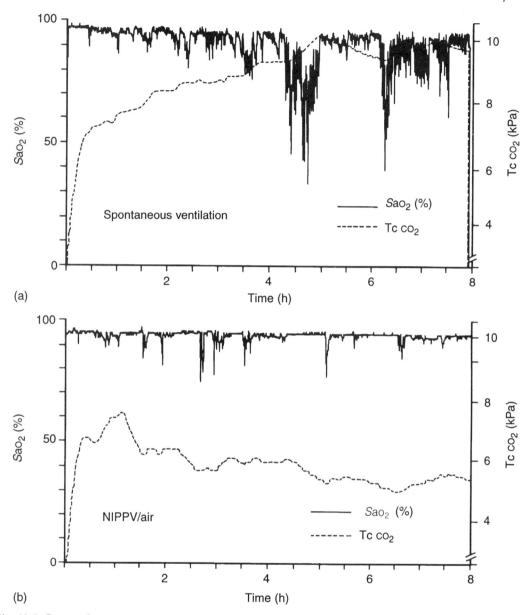

Fig. 12.7 Overnight monitoring of arterial oxygen saturation (——) and transcutaneous CO_2 (---) and in an adolescent with Duchenne muscular dystrophy: (a) at presentation with symptoms of severe nocturnal hypoventilation; (b) the following night while receiving NIPPV.

REFERENCES

1. Adams, A.B., Whitman, J. and Marcy, T. (1993) Surveys of long-term ventilatory support in Minnesota: 1986 and 1992. *Chest*, **103**, 1463–9.
2. Robinson, R.O. (1990) Ventilator dependency in the United Kingdom. *Arch. Dis. Childh.*, **65**, 1235–6.
3. Melki, J., Abdelhak, S., Sheth, P. *et al.* (1990) Gene for chronic proximal spinal muscular atrophies maps to chromosome 5 q. *Nature*, **344**, 767–8.
4. Barois, A. and Estournet-Mathiaud, B. (1992) Ventilatory support at home in children with spinal muscular atrophies (SMA). *Eur. Respir. Rev.*, **10**, 319–22.
5. Rideau, Y., Gatin, G., Bach, J. and Gines, G. (1983) Prolongation of life in Duchenne's muscular dystrophy. *Acta. Neurol.*, **5**, 118–24.
6. Baydur, A., Gilgoff, I., Prentice, W. *et al.* (1990) Decline in respiratory function and experience with long term assisted ventilation in advanced Duchenne's muscular dystrophy. *Chest*, **97**, 884–9.
7. Nigro, G., Coni, L.I., Politano, L. and Bain, R.J.I. (1990) The incidence and evolution of cardiomyopthy in Duchenne muscular dystrophy. *Int. J. Cardiol.*, **26**, 271–7.
8. Barbe, F., Quera-Salva, M.A., McCann, C. *et al.* (1994) Sleep-related respiratory disturbances in patients with Duchenne muscular dystrophy. *Eur. Respir. J.*, **7**, 1403–8.
9. Khan, Y. and Heckmatt, J.Z. (1994) Obstructive apnoeas in Duchenne muscular dystrophy. *Thorax*, **49**, 157–61.
10. Alexander, M.A., Johnson, E.W., Petty, J. and Stauch, D. (1979) Mechanical ventilation of patients with late stage Duchenne muscular dystrophy: management in the home. *Arch. Phys. Med. Rehabil.*, **60**, 289–92.
11. Hill, N.S., Redline, S., Carskadon, M. *et al.* (1992) Sleep-disordered breathing in patients with Duchenne muscular dystrophy using negative pressure ventilators. *Chest*, **102**, 1656–62.
12. Bach, J.R., O'Brien, J., Krotenberg, R. and Alba, A.S. (1987) Management of end stage respiratory failure in Duchenne muscular dystrophy. *Muscle and Nerve*, **10**, 177–82.
13. Heckmatt, J.Z., Loh, L. and Dubowitz, V. (1990) Night-time nasal ventilation in neuromuscular disease. *Lancet*, **335**, 579–82.
14. Ellis, E.R., Bye, P.T.B., Bruderer, J.W. and Sullivan, C.E. (1987) Treatment of respiratory failure during sleep in patients with neuromuscular disease. *Am. Rev. Respir. Dis.*, **135**, 148–52.
15. Raphael, J-C., Chevret, S., Chastang, C., Bouvet, F. (The French Multicentric Group) (1992) A prospective multicentre study of home mechanical ventilation in Duchenne de Boulogne muscular dystrophy. *Eur. Respir. Rev.*, **2**, 312–16.
16. Vianello, A., Bevilacqua, M., Salvador, V. *et al.* (1994) Long-term nasal intermittent positive pressure ventilation in advanced Duchenne's Muscular Dystrophy. *Chest*, **105**, 445–8.
17. Hill, N.S. (1994) Noninvasive positive pressure ventilation in neuromuscular disease. Enough is enough. *Chest*, **105**, 337–8.
18. Smith, P.E.M., Calverley, P.M.A., Edwards, R.H.T. *et al.* (1987) Practical problems in the respiratory care of patients with muscular dystrophy. *N. Engl. J. Med.*, **316**, 1197–205.
19. Raphael, J-C., Chevret, S., Chastang, C. and Bouvet, F. (1994) Randomised trial of preventive nasal ventilation in Duchenne muscular dystrophy. *Lancet*, **343**, 1600–4.
20. Muntoni, F., Hird, M. and Simonds, A.K. (1994) Preventative nasal ventilation in Duchenne muscular dystrophy (Letter). *Lancet*, **344**, 340.
21. Dubowitz, V. (1989) *A Colour Atlas of Muscle Disorders in Childhood*. Wolfe Medical Publications, London.
22. Barois, A. and Estournet-Mathiaud, B. (1993) Nasal ventilation in congenital myopathies and spinal muscular atrophies. *Eur. Respir. Rev.*, **3**, 12, 275–8.
23. Ras, G.J., Van Staden, M., Schultz, C. *et al.* (1994) Respiratory manifestations of rigid spine syndrome. *Am. J. Respir. Crit. Care. Med.*, **150**, 540–6.
24. Colver, A.F., Steer, C.R., Godman, M.J. and Uttley, W.S. (1981) Rigid spine syndrome and fatal cardiomyopathy. *Arch. Dis. Childh.*, **56**, 148–51.

114

25. Aday, L.H., Wegener, D.H., Anderson, R.M. and Aitken, M.J. (1989) Home care for ventilator-assisted children. *Health Affairs*, Summer, 137–47.

26. Lantos, J.D. and Kohrman, A.F. (1992) Ethical aspects of pediatric home care. *Pediatrics*, **89**, 920–4.

13

Continuous positive airway pressure therapy

ANITA K. SIMONDS

INTRODUCTION

Continuous positive airway pressure (CPAP) therapy was introduced as a treatment for obstructive sleep spnoea (OSA) by Sullivan and colleagues in 1981 [1]. It has revolutionized the approach to this condition, virtually abolishing the need for tracheostomy which was previously recommended for severe OSA. CPAP can also be used in patients with acute hyoxaemia due to conditions such as pneumonia, pulmonary oedema and exacerbations of COPD, and may be effective in some adults and infants with central sleep apnoea. As a major application is in obstructive sleep apnoea, this use will be covered in detail. Alternative approaches including upper airway surgery and pharmacological measures will be compared and contrasted with CPAP.

SLEEP APNOEA SYNDROMES

An apnoeic episode is defined as 10 seconds or more of cessation of airflow at the nose and mouth. The apnoea is obstructive in origin if respiratory effort occurs throughout the apnoea, and central if there is no accompanying respiratory effort. Episodes of reduction in airflow (>10 seconds) are called hypopnoeas; exact definitions vary from laboratory to laboratory. The syndrome of obstructive sleep apnoea can be described as multiple episodes of apnoea or hyponoea associated with clinical impairment, e.g. increased somnolence or altered cardiopulmonary function. Somnolence arises as apnoeic/hypopnoiec episodes are terminated by arousal, and in the presence of multiple arousals sleep becomes fragmented and unrefreshing. Long-term OSA is associated with an increase in mortality and morbidity from vascular events including myocardial infarction and stroke [2]. Most workers in the field would agree that a spectrum exists which extends from simple snoring, through symptomatic snoring to the obstructive sleep apnoea syndrome. The presence of more than 15 apnoeas and hyponoeas per hour (apnoea/hypopnoea index, AHI) during sleep is usually regarded as abnormal, but of greater importance than AHI is the physiological impact on sleep quality, arterial oxygen desaturation and cardiovascular function. Snoring in the absence of apnoeas or desaturation can fragment sleep and cause somnolence, this condition is known as the upper airways resistance syndrome [3]. It is

Non-Invasive Respiratory Support. Edited by Anita Simonds. Published by Chapman & Hall, London. ISBN 0412 56840 3.

important to note that the criteria used to diagnose and quantify OSA in children differ from those used for adults [4]. This is partly because significant desaturation can occur in children with episodes lasting less than 10 seconds.

A prevalence study [5] of adults aged 30–60 years in the USA showed that OSA with an AHI >15 was present in 9% of males and 4% of females; symptoms related to sleep disordered breathing were reported in 4% of males and 2% of females. In a UK study [6] of sleep disordered breathing 1% of men had more than 10 dips in arterial oxygen saturation/hour. OSA is therefore a common condition and an increasing number of patients requiring treatment are likely to be seen. The common presenting features include snoring, apnoeas witnessed by partner, hypersomnolence and nocturnal choking. The assessment and investigation of patients with suspected OSA has been reviewed recently [7]. Snoring, obstructive sleep apnoea and central sleep apnoea can be distinguished by overnight monitoring of respiration (sleep study).

Oximetry alone lacks sufficient sensitivity and specificity to be adequate as a screening investigation of OSA. Polysomnography (Table 13.1) is the gold standard investigation, but is demanding in technician time and cost. Early data suggest that limited multichannel monitoring which includes assessment of snoring, airflow respiratory effort and oxygenation may be a practical substitute for conventional polysomnography for clinical purposes. Suitable alternatives are video/oximetry/snoring systems or monitoring of nasal flow profile/snoring and oximetry. Polysomnography should be available for cases in which limited multichannel screening produces equivocal results, or when sleep –wake disorders other than OSA are suspected, e.g. narcolepsy, benign idiopathic hypersomnolence. A suggested approach to investigation is given in Table 13.2.

Table 13.1 Polysomnography

Channel	Data
Electroencephalogram (EEG)	Arousals
Electro-oculogram (EOG)	Sleep stages
Electromyogram (EMG)	Non REM 1–4
	REM
	Wake
Pulse oximetry	Arterial oxygen saturation
	Heart rate
Airflow at nose and mouth	
+	Characterization of apnoeas
	Apnoea/hypopnoea index
Rib cage and abdominal movement	
Microphone/decibel meter	Snoring
Position monitor	Posture in bed
Leg movement	Periodic leg movement

Table 13.2 Which type of sleep study?

Category	Monitoring
High probability OSA	Limited multichannel study. If negative result, proceed to polysomnography
Low probability OSA	Limited multichannel study at hospital or home
Possibility of non-respiratory sleep/wake disorder (e.g. narcolepsy) *or* Equivocal result in screening study	Polysomnography
Parasomnia	Video multichannel system or Polysomnography
At-risk patient Nocturnal hypoventilation	Oximetry and $TcCO_2$ monitoring $+/-$ multichannel screening study
Titration of CPAP treatment	Multichannel screening study at hospital or home *or* CPAP 'autoset' machine
Titration of assisted ventilation/O_2 therapy	Oximetry and $TcCO_2$

PATHOPHYSIOLOGY AND MECHANISM OF ACTION IN OSA

During sleep the patency of the upper airway is preserved by a balance between forces predisposing to airway collapse and those responsible for actively dilating the airway (Fig. 13.1).

Dynamic viewing of the airway during sleep using fluouroscopy [8] has shown that airway collapse commonly begins in the oropharyngeal region, progressing to the hypopharynx or laryngopharynx. The soft palate is pulled down as a plug into the oropharynx in many patients. Endoscopic visualization during sleep [9] has confirmed that airway collapse occurs in a number of regions either simultaneously or progressively. In this study of 45 patients the following patterns were seen: primary narrowing at the level of the nasopharnyx plus other sites of secondary narrowing in 40%; primary narrowing in the nasopharynx plus other sites of primary narrowing in 22%; and primary narrowing only in the nasopharynx in 18%. Other combinations of collapse were seen in the remaining patients.

CPAP exerts its effect by splinting the upper airway open throughout its length. Additional benefits include an increase in functional residual capacity and a reduction in the inspiratory work of breathing. In each case the level of continuous positive pressure needs to be titrated to the individual, to achieve maximum benefit (Fig. 13.2)

INDICATIONS IN OSA/UPPER AIRWAY RESISTANCE SYNDROME

CPAP (Fig. 13.3) can be effective therpay for all forms of OSA and the upper airway resistance syndrome. The decision to start

118

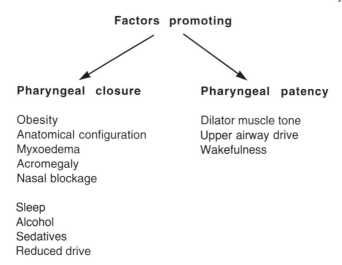

Fig. 13.1 Factors resposible for promoting upper airway collapse and maintaining patency.

CPAP is dependent on the severity of the effects of the sleep disordered breathing and the feasibility of the suitable alternative measures discussed below.

The diagnosis of OSA should be established by monitoring of breathing during sleep as described above. In particular daytime hypersomnolence is a key indication for intervention. Hypersomnolence can be quantitated subjectively using questionnaires such as the Epworth Sleepiness Scale [10] (Fig. 13.4) or Stanford Sleepiness Scale [11]. The median sleep latency time (MLST) can be established using polysomnography and offers a quantitative measure, although not all UK sleep laboratories offer this facility routinely. In practice, hypersomnolence can be described as falling asleep inappropriately during the day in spite of a normal duration of nocturnal sleep [11]. Sleepiness when driving is a particular concern, in view of the increased incidence of road traffic accidents in OSA patients [12]. The presence of significant desaturation or cardiovascular complications such as nocturnal dysrrhythmias and angina, and uncontrolled hypertension should lower the threshold for instituting CPAP.

Reversible causes of OSA include obesity and endocrine disorders such as hypothyroidism and acromegaly. If OSA is severe, CPAP can be used while the patient loses weight or until endocrine treatment has taken effect. Hormone replacement therapy may have a role in postmenopausal female patients, but is unlikely to effect a cure [13].

Standards for the use of CPAP in sleep apnoea syndromes have been set recently by the American Thoracic Society [14].

UPPER AIRWAY SURGERY

Nasal surgery

Optimizing the nasal airway by correcting a deviated septum, removal of polyps or treating rhinitis will decrease upstream resistance, thereby reducing the tendency to pharyngeal collapse. These measures should be considered in individuals with symptomatic nasal blockage. However, as the main level of airway obstruction is usually in the pharynx, nasal surgery may reduce snoring and modify OSA, but rarely abolishes the condition. In individuals with structural nasal

119

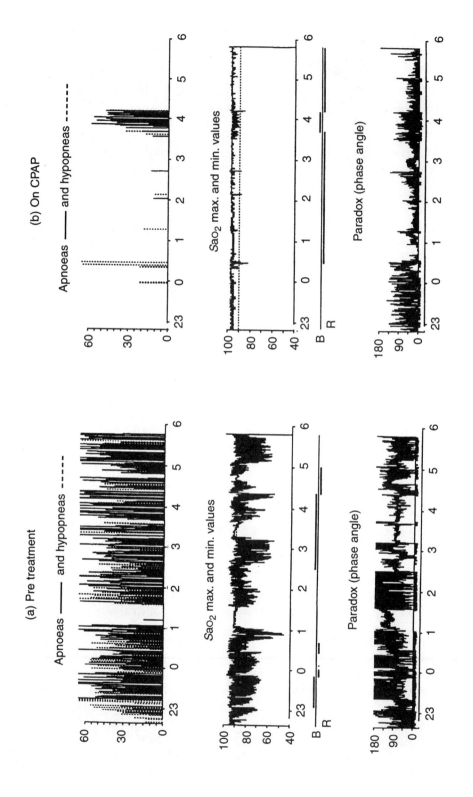

Fig. 13.2 Sleep study data demonstrating (A) obstructive sleep apnoea with (B) Response to CPAP. Some residual apnoeas are seen around 4 a.m.

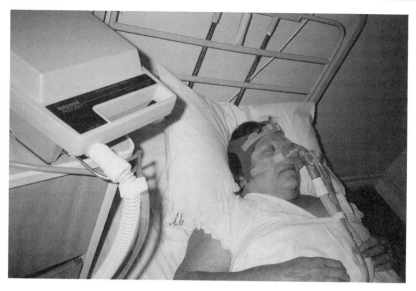

Fig. 13.3 Continuous positive airway pressure therapy.

airway obstruction surgical attention may faciliate the use of CPAP.

Tonsillectomy and adenoidectomy

Enlargement of tonsils (+/− adenoidal tissue) is the commonest cause of upper airway obstruction in children with sleep apnoea and can easily be visualized on examination. Lymphoid growth is maximal at the age of around 5 years, but occasionally tonsils remain hypertrophied in adolescence and young adulthood rather than regressing. Tonsillectomy in this situation is usually helpful regardless of age [15].

Uvulopalatopharyngoplasty (UVPP)

This procedure was pioneered by Fujita in 1981 and usually includes resection of the uvula, part of the soft palate and pharnyx. The aim is to improve the airway and stiffen it so that collapse during sleep is resisted. Many patients are attracted by the possibility of a once and for all cure to the problem

of OSA, rather than a lifetime of CPAP. However, the outcome of UVPP is difficult to interpret as surgical technique can vary from surgeon to surgeon, and not all subjects have undergone long-term polysomnographic follow-up. Although some centres have reported early benefit, evidence suggests that in a proportion of patients subjective reduction in snoring is not accompanied by a marked decrease in apnoea/hypopnoea index. Indeed the decrease in snoring may mask continued severe obstructive episodes. In addition, UVPP may be complicated by palatal incompetence and pharyngeal stenosis. Late results can also be disappointing, although a recent study [16] which compared UVPP and CPAP in patients with mild or moderate OSA showed no difference in long-term survival between the two treatments. This finding contrasts with results from an earlier study [17] which showed increased mortality in UVPP patients.

In view of these problems attempts have been made to select the patients most likely to respond to UVPP [18,19]. Launois *et al.* [20]

121

Epworth Sleepiness Scale

This scale assesses your level of sleepiness during the day.

How likely are you to doze off or fall asleep in the following situations, in contrast to felling just tired? This refers to your usual way of life in recent times. Even if you have not done some of these things recently try to work out how they would have affected you. Use the following scale to choose the *most appropriate number* for each situation.

    0 = would ***never*** doze   **1** = ***slight*** chance of dozing
    2 = ***moderate*** chance of dozing   **3** = ***high*** chance of dozing

SITUATION	CHANCE OF DOZING
Sitting and reading	....
Watching TV	....
Sitting, inactive in a public place (e.g. theatre or a meeting)	....
As a passenger in a car for an hour without a break	....
Lying down for a rest in the afternoon when circumstances permit	....
Sitting and talking to someone	....
Sitting quietly after a lunch without alcohol	....
In a car, while stopped for a few minutes in the traffic	....

Fig. 13.4 Epworth Sleepiness Scale. (Reproduced from Johns [10]).

suggest that individuals with airway collapse at nasopharyngeal level, without secondary areas of collapse elsewhere, are the best candidates for UVPP. Airway compromise at hypopharyngeal level is unlikely to respond to UVPP, as surgery is carried out rostral to this site.

Laser-assisted uvulopalatoplasty (LAUP)

This procedure differs from conventional UVPP in that laser application to the soft palate is used to shorten the palate and uvula with the aim of reducing vibration of these structures and, hence, snoring. The lateral pharyngeal wall and tonsils are not involved in the procedure. Therapy is often given over several sessions. Kamami [21] has reported that snoring was eliminated or reduced in 77.4% of 34 patients who underwent laser-assisted uvulopalatoplasty. However, it should be stressed that there are no peer-reviewed outcome data on the results of LAUP for snoring and no evidence whatsover that it has a role in the management of OSA. In view of the controversy surrounding LAUP, the American Sleep Disorders Association has produced a series of recommendations on the topic [22]. These suggest that LAUP should *not* be recommended in OSA. Candidates with snoring should be evaluated with monitoring of respiration during sleep to exclude OSA. Patients should be informed that the benefits, risks and side-effects of LAUP have not yet been established. When used in snorers, LAUP may delay the subsequent diagnosis of OSA, by removing the warning feature of snoring. As with conventional UVPP, care should be taken when prescribing sedatives or sedative analgesia to individuals undergoing upper airway surgery.

UVPP versus CPAP

There is persuasive evidence showing that CPAP is preferable to UVPP in severe OSA. The situation in less severe cases is not as clear. While it is important not to be prescriptive, our practice is to use CPAP as the treatment of choice in moderate or severe OSA, especially when somnolence is marked (Epworth sleepiness score >12), AHI exceeds 30 and/or episodes are associated with hypoxaemia and cardiovascular stress. Individuals with severe snoring alone, or snoring and mild OSA undergo full airway assessment including sleep nasendoscopy. If this indicates nasopharyngeal airway compromise the advantages and disadvantages of surgery are discussed with the patient. Patients treated with surgery for OSA undergo

a sleep study after the procedure and continue long-term follow-up. Further studies comparing CPAP with UVPP in patients with mild OSA are urgently needed.

It has been suggested that CPAP treatment cannot be used effectively in patients who have undergone UVPP. We have not found this to be the case, although the extent of the surgery is clearly an important factor.

Maxillofacial surgery

A complex staged surgical approach to OSA has been developed at Stanford, USA. Here, maxillo-mandibular advancement is used to enlarge the pharynx. Results from this centre are encouraging [23], but have not been duplicated widely. At present this type of radical surgery is advisable only in those with severe facial disproportion.

Tracheostomy

Bypassing the upper airway by tracheostomy abolishes obstructive episodes, but is associated with considerable morbidity in its own right and imposes significant social limitations on the patient. Any additional central apnoea component may not be adequately treated with a tracheostomy alone. Since the advent of CPAP, a formal tracheostomy for OSA is rarely needed. Minitracheostomy has been used as a temporizing measure [24], but the stoma is probably too small for effective ventilation.

Oronasal prostheses

Any device which pulls the tongue base forward during sleep might have a role is treating patients with obstruction at this level. A worthwhile reduction in apnoea/hypopnoea index has been demonstrated using a removable mandibular advancement device and this was well tolerated [25]. These devices require further assessment.

The Nozovent is a nasal dilator which has

been advocated to reduce snoring. Hoffstein *et al.* [26] have shown that its effect on snoring is trivial, although some individuals claim benefit. There is no evidence that it is effective in OSA.

PHARMACOLOGICAL TREATMENT

Although a number of drug treatments have been recommended for OSA, including medroxyprogesterone and strychnine, the only agent that produces a significant improvement in nocturnal oxygenation and AHI is protriptyline. This non-sedative tricyclic drug appears to act by reducing REM-sleep related sleep disordered breathing [27], and may have an independent action on upper airway tone [28]. A mild benefical effect in snoring has also been demonstrated [29]. However, anticholinergic side-effects are common, and doses above 10 mg at night are poorly tolerated. Protriptyline may be worth trying in patients with mild REM related OSA. It should be avoided where possible in patients with prostatism, as urinary retention can be precipitated. Impotence and constipation are other relatively frequent complaints.

EFFECTS OF CPAP IN OSA

When established correctly, CPAP immediately controls sleep disordered breathing and rapidly reduces daytime somnolence [30]. Retrospective analysis shows that long-term CPAP lessens morbidity and mortality due to OSA [17].

INDICATIONS IN CENTRAL SLEEP APNOEA

Central sleep apnoea can be divided into two categories: patients with alveolar hypoventilation due to impaired chemosensitivity, and those with increased respiratory drive. It is the latter group which may respond to CPAP therapy. This includes individuals with periodic (Cheyne–Stokes) respiration due to cardiac failure. In some of these patients symptoms of sleep fragmentation *and* cardiac function may improve with the introduction of CPAP therapy [31]. However, CPAP may worsen symptoms in occasional patients with severe left ventricular dysfunction and so this treatment should only be used with careful monitoring and follow-up.

CPAP may also have a role in neonates with apnoea syndromes. This work is at an early stage and there are few controlled data available.

ROLE IN ACUTE HYPOXAEMIC LUNG DISEASE

CPAP has an established role in treating refractory hypoxaemia in patients with acute pulmonary oedema [32] and severe pneumonia [33]. The treatment works by increasing alveolar recruitment and functional residual capacity, decreasing anatomical shunting, and reducing the work of breathing. In these acute situations CPAP therapy is generally provided on an intensive care unit or high dependency ward using demand flow generator systems supplied with a piped oxygen/air blender. CPAP in acute COPD is discussed elsewhere (Chapters 4 and 6).

CHOICE OF EQUIPMENT FOR DOMICILIARY USE

A wide range of portable CPAP systems is available. As described above, the CPAP unit is a flow generator which should be capable of delivering a constant pressure throughout the respiratory cycle. Ideally, it should be reliable, portable, inexpensive and function as noiselessly as possible. Systems cost between £400 and £800. Several studies comparing different devices show that there is little to choose between them in performance characteristics [34]. For this reason cost is often the main determinant in purchasing the equipment.

Many machines provide a gradual ramped increase in CPAP to the preset level in the first 5–20 minutes of use. Some individuals, particularly those beginning treatment or those who require high CPAP levels, find this helpful. Others find the ramp unnecessary and prefer to 'get on with' the predetermined pressure as soon as the mask is in place. We do not routinely provide humidification, but this may be indicated in some patients, as described below.

MASK SELECTION

This is discussed in Chapter 3. Nasal pillows or plugs (Adam circuit, Puritan Bennett) are as efficient at delivering CPAP as a nasal mask [35]. If the patient is severely hypersomnolent or confused mouth leaks will reduce the efficiency of treatment; here a full facemask is recommended. These masks have a quick release mechanism to reduce the risk of aspiration in an obtunded patient, although clearly such a patient would require close observation. Individialized masks or nosepieces can be constructed for patients who cannot be adequately fitted with an 'off the peg' mask.

STARTING CPAP

As with any new treatment, the aim and principles of CPAP therapy should be explained to the patient. Starting pressures of between 5 and 10 cm H_2O are usual, although some individuals require higher values. Several centres have developed algorithms to predict the pressure level required, but these have not always been validated prospectively. Engelman and colleagues [36] have shown that the most important factors determining CPAP pressure are collar size and apnoea/hypopnoea index, which together explained

53% of the variance in prescribed CPAP levels.

It is often helpful first to try CPAP during an afternoon nap, so that any early problems can be identified and solved before nocturnal monitoring. Acclimatization rates are very variable. The more somnolent the patient the more likely he/she is to tolerate the treatment and therefore a CPAP titration study may be feasible on the first night of treatment. Others find they sleep poorly using CPAP at first and so an early titration study may be unrepresentative.

CPAP TITRATION

Conventional CPAP titration studies require the technician to be present all night to carry out polysomnography and adjust CPAP level until obstructive episodes and their consequences are abolished. As the degree of sleep fragmentation and number of arousals determines the degree of daytime somnolence, ideally CPAP should reduce arousals to a minimum. This requires EEG, EOG and EMG monitoring which adds to the cost of the study, and is not available in all centres. However, autonomic phenomena such as change in heart rate and blood pressure seem to reflect arousals accurately and can be more easily monitored [37].

'INTELLIGENT' (AUTOSETTING) CPAP

It is likely that 'intelligent' CPAP machines (e.g. Rescare Ltd., DeVilbiss) will become used increasingly to establish patients on CPAP. These machines detect flow in the mask and automatically adjust CPAP until normal flow is restored (Fig. 13.5). Safeguards are incorporated so that the CPAP level is not increased in response to central apnoeas. These autoset systems obviate the need for a technician to be in attendance overnight and make it easier for titration studies to be carried out at home. The long-term benefits

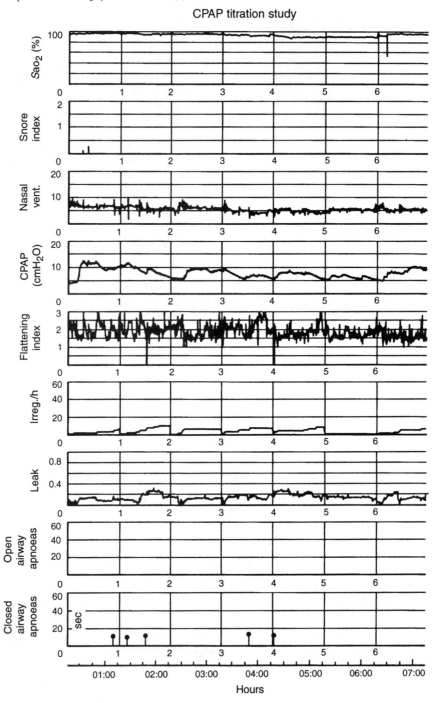

Fig. 13.5 Autoset titration of CPAP. CPAP level (fourth bar from the top) varies to normalize nasal ventilation.

of autoset systems compared to conventional CPAP titration are being examined. The Sullivan Autoset Clinical system (Rescare Ltd) can be used in diagnostic and CPAP titration mode.

CPAP OR BiPAP?

The majority of patients with OSA are normocapnic by day and show no evidence of marked nocturnal CO_2 retention. CPAP is usually sufficient to control desaturation in these individuals. It has been postulated that the availability of two levels of pressure with the BiPAP mechine may increase patient comfort and improve compliance over CPAP alone. However, in practive similar levels of compliance are seen (CPAP 74%, BiPAP 77% in a 6-month follow-up study [38]). BiPAP does have a role, however, in hypercapnic patients. These usually present with a combination of OSA plus COPD, massive obesity or respiratory muscle weakness. By improving minute ventilation BiPAP enhances CO_2 clearance, and reduces the work of breathing more effectively than CPAP [39]. In some individuals with severe end-stage OSA complicated by respiratory failure and cor pulmonale, BiPAP may be used in hospital intensively to rapidly correct arterial blood tensions. Once stability has been achieved it may be possible to switch to CPAP for maintenance therapy at home.

COMPLIANCE

Compliance with CPAP therapy is determined by a number of features, the most important being the trade-off between symptom improvement and side-effects as experienced by the patient. Compliance has been assessed subjectively and objectively.

Hoffstein and colleagues [40] used a questionnaire to assess the pattern of CPAP use and side-effects in 148 subjects. Response rate was 65%. Seventy per cent of subjects

prescribed CPAP continued using it, with 81% believing it to be an effective treatment. Around 60% felt more awake during the day, and snoring was reported to be improved or eradicated by 76 patients. Seventeen patients were unable to persist with treatment. Interestingly, the side-effects in these patients did not differ from those who continued CPAP – the chief problems being claustrophobia, nasal discomfort and the nuisance of having to use the equipment every night. In most of the failed users, a marked improvement in AHI was obtained, so compliance did not clearly correspond to the efficiency of treatment. An ANTADIR study [41] of 193 patients in France showed that 88% reported CPAP use for an average of 6.5 ± 3 hours a night, with only 1% claiming no benefit. Fifty per cent had side-effects, mainly related to the mask.

Reported use by patients is likely to overestimate compliance. Kribbs *et al*, [42] have examined this issue objectively using hidden microprocessor time clocks. In this study although 60% of patients claimed to use CPAP every night, monitoring showed that only 46% used the treatment for at least 4 hours per night for 70% of the days studied. Those using CPAP regularly tended to be more hypersomnolent at the start of treatment and experience greater benefit with use. The commonest complaints were inconvenience and nasal stuffiness.

Confirmatory data from the Edinburgh group [36] suggest that, despite intensive encouragement, their patients use CPAP for only 4.7 hours at night. There was no correlation between CPAP use and improvement in multiple sleep latency or apnoea/hypopnoea index. Reeves-Hoche *et al.* [43] have shown a similar level of use (mean 4.2 hours/night), and found no factors that would predict the likelihood of good or poor compliance, although there was a tendency for poor compliers to have an increased number of CPAP side-effects.

Overall, these studies would suggest that CPAP therapy needs to become much more user-friendly. Prompt attention to side-effects and practical problems, improved mask design and accurate titration of CPAP setting may all improve the acceptability of treatment.

PRACTICAL PROBLEMS

NASAL STUFFINESS/RHINITIS

It is suggested that nasal congestion or streaming may be most marked in patients with hyperresponsiveness to cold air, but this has not been confirmed. In individuals with occasional nasal obstruction at the time of an upper respiratory tract infection, ephedrine 0.5% nasal drops for a short period are usually effective. Frequent use of ephedrine should be discouraged as this may lead to rebound nasal congestion. Patients with a history of perennial or seasonal rhinitis should undergo a trial of nasal corticosteroid.

Nasal streaming may respond to ipratroprium nasal spray or a combination of ipratropium and nasal corticosteroid.

An alternative approach is to add humidification (Fig. 13.6).

MASK DISCOMFORT

See Chapter 5.

CLAUSTROPHOBIA

This is often an early problem and usually responds to encouragement and support. The nasal plugs cover less of the face and may be helpful in this situation. A continued sensation of claustrophia and a feeling of suffocation should prompt a check on the CPAP setting, as this may be inadequate or too high.

MOUTH LEAKS

See Chapter 5.

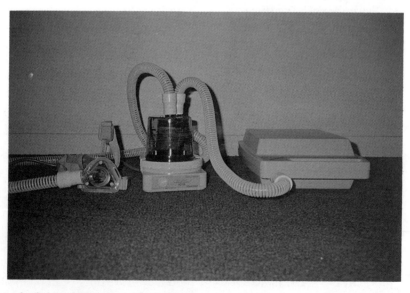

Fig. 13.6 Water bath humidification with CPAP.

NOISE

Sound levels are similar in most systems [34] and most bed partners find the sound of the CPAP machine preferable to snoring. Some patients place the machines outside the bedroom door to reduce noise levels. This is acceptable providing CPAP levels at the mask are maintained.

COST/FUNDING OF CPAP EQUIPMENT
(SEE CHAPTER 15)

In some areas of the UK CPAP machines are not available on the National Health Service. This has caused severe problems in some centres with patients deprived of an effective treatment, and some individuals having to pay for their machine. This is inequitable. The Royal College of Physicians report on Sleep Apnoea and related conditions [11] strongly advises that purchasers should make adequate provision for funding of equipment, and also ensure that sufficient facilities for sleep studies are available in their region. No NHS patient should have to buy a CPAP machine if full investigation proves this treatment is indicated.

Problems also exist in funding private sleep studies, in that some insurance companies will cover this investigation while others do not. This is anomalous, and in view of the health risk that untreated OSA poses, does not make good sense. Some companies (e.g. BUPA) request completion of a standard symptom questionnaire by a specialist before sanctioning investigation for OSA. Funding of CPAP and ventilatory equipment in Europe is discussed in Chapter 16.

COMMON QUESTIONS FROM PATIENTS

1. Should CPAP be used every night?

Many patients experiment with CPAP use to answer this question themselves. During the first night off CPAP after a period of effective use, symptoms are usually improved compared to pre-treatment levels, probably due to the reduction in sleep deprivation. Reduction in pharyngeal oedema will also enhance airway calibre. After several nights, symptoms and sleep disordered breathing return. In patients who lose a significant amount of weight, or who receive effective treatment for endocrine disorders, or upper airway surgery, a repeat sleep study should be carried out to determine whether CPAP therapy is still needed.

2. What arrangements should be made for service and maintenance of equipment?

CPAP machines should be serviced once a year. Manufacturer's instructions should be observed. The service is a simple procedure and may be carried out locally or the machine sent away to the dealer, although the latter is less acceptable. Filters should be changed regularly according to the manufacturer's guide. Silicone nasal masks should last for 6–12 months if they are well cared for.

3. What arrangements should be made for taking CPAP equipment abroad?

During airflights CPAP equiment should be transported by hand as cabin luggage. Carry holdalls are available for most CPAP models or these can be bought off the peg (Fig. 13.7). Patients should take with them a report stating CPAP requirements. In addition to health insurance cover, arrangements should be made regarding insurance of the equipment depending on whether the machine is on loan or belongs to the patient. It is important to ensure that there will be no problems with voltage incompatibility in the country to be visited. Some CPAP machines operate with dual voltage (220/110) and are convenient for patients visiting the USA. For travellers in Europe, centres participating

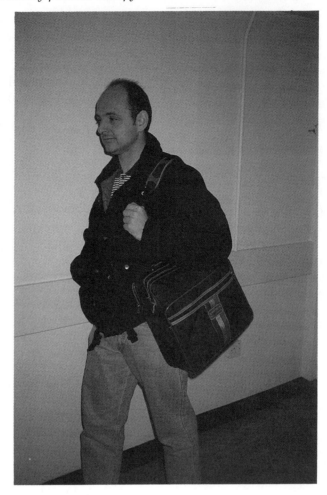

Fig. 13.7 CPAP carry case for ease of travel.

in the Eurolung Assistance Scheme [44] may be able to help in the event of equipment problems.

4. Driving and OSA

As indicated above, individuals with OSA are at risk of being involved in road traffic accidents as a result of lapses in concentration and falling asleep at the wheel. This risk may be as much as ten times that of the normal population. The Medical Advisory Branch of the Driver and Vehicle Licensing Agency (DVLA) recommend that driving should cease if excessive sleepiness is present. Driving is permitted once satisfactory control of symptoms is achieved. It is the duty of the licence holder to inform the DVLA if his/her condition poses a risk to driving [5]. Vocational drivers (Schedule 2) of large goods vehicles or passenger carrying vehicles (LGV/PCV), formally known as HGV/PSV drivers, who have a confirmed diagnosis of OSA, should cease driving. Driving may be resumed subject to review when it is confirmed by a specialist that the condition has been adequately controlled for at least 12 months (DVLA, Update 1993). Drivers should be clearly informed of the risks of somnulence and driving and their responsibility for reporting OSA.

REFERENCES

1. Sullivan, C.E., Berthon Jones, M. and Issa, F.G. (1981) Reversal of obstructive sleep apnoea by continuous positive airway pressure applied through the nares. *Lancet*, **1**, 862–5.
2. Stradling, J.R. (1993) Longer term consequences of sleep apnoea, in *Handbook of Sleep Related Breathing Disorders*, Oxford University Press, Oxford, pp. 56–64.
3. Guilleminault, C., Stoohs, R., Clerk, A. *et al.* (1993) A cause of excessive sleepiness. The upper airway resistance syndrome. *Chest*, **104**, 781–7.
4. Rosen, C.L., D'Andrea, L. and Haddad, G.G. (1992) Adult criteria for obstructive sleep apnea do not identify children with serious obstruction. *Am. Rev. Respir. Dis.*, **146**, 1231–4.
5. Young, T., Palta, M., Dempsey, J. *et al.* (1993) The occurrence of sleep disordered breathing among middle-aged adults. *N. Engl. J. Med.*, **328**, 1230–5.
6. Stradling, J.R. and Crosby, J.H. (1991) Predictors and prevalence of obstructive sleep apnoea and snoring in 1001 middle aged men. *Thorax*, 46, 85–90.
7. Simonds, A.K. (1994) Sleep studies of respiratory function and home respiratory support. *Br. Med. J.*, **309**, 35–40.
8. Pepin, J.L., Ferretti, G., Veale, D. *et al.* (1992) Somnofluoroscopy, computed tomography and cephalometry in the assessment of the airway in obstructive sleep apnoea. *Thorax*, **47**, 150–6.
9. Morrison, D.L., Launois, S.H., Isono, S. *et al.* (1993) Pharyngeal narrowing and closing pressures in patients with obstructive sleep apnea. *Am. Rev. Respir. Dis.*, **148**, 606–11.
10. Johns, M.W. (1991) A new method for measuring daytime sleepiness: the Epworth sleepiness scale. *Sleep*, **14**, 540–5.
11. Royal College of Physicians (1993) Report: Sleep apnoea and related conditions. London, RCP.
12. Findley, L.J., Unversagt, M.E. and Surratt, P.M. (1988) Automobile accidents involving patients with obstructive apnea. *Am. Rev. Respir. Dis.*, **138**, 337–40.
13. Cistulli, P.A., Barnes, D.J., Grunstein, R.R. and Sullivan, C.E. (1994) Effect of short term hormone replacement therpay in postmenopausal women with obstructive sleep apnea. *Thorax*, **49**, 699–702.
14. American Thoracic Society (1994) Indications and standards for use of nasal continuous positive airway pressure (CPAP) in sleep apnea syndromes. *Am. J. Respir. Crit. Care Med.*, **150**, 1738–45.
15. Kryger, M.H. (1994) Management of obstructive sleep apnea: overview, in *Principles and Practice of Sleep Medicine* (eds M.H. Kryger, T. Roth and W.C. Dement), 2nd edn, W.B. Saunders, Philadelphia, p. 741.
16. Keenan, S.P., Burt, H., Ryan, F. and Fleetham, J.A. (1994) Long-term survival of patients with obstructive sleep apnoea treated by uvulopalatopharyngoplasty or nasal CPAP. *Chest*, **105**, 155–9.
17. He, J., Krygen, M., Zorich, F. *et al.* (1988) Mortality and apnea index in obstructive sleep apnea. *Chest*, **94**, 9–14.
18. Sher, A.E., Thorpy, M.J., Shprintzen, R.J. *et al.* (1985) Predictive value of the Mueller maneuver in selection of patients for uvulopalatopharyngoplasty. *Laryngoscope*, **95**, 1483–7.
19. Katsantonis, G.P., Maas, C.S. and Walsh, J.K. (1989) The predictive efficacy of the Mueller maneuver in uvulopalatopharyngoplasty. *Laryngoscope*, **99**, 677–80.
20. Launois, S.H., Feroah, T.R., Campbell, W.N. (1993) Site of pharyngeal narrowing predicts outcome of surgery for obstructive sleep apnea. *Am. Rev. Respir. Dis.*, **149**, 182–9.
21. Kamami, Y.V. (1990) Laser CO_2 for snoring. Preliminary results. *Acta Otorhinolaryngol. Belg.*, **44**, 451–6.
22. American Sleep Disorders Association Report (1994) Practice parameters for use of laser-assisted uvulopalatoplasty. *Sleep*, **17**, 744–8.
23. Riley, R.W., Powell, N.B. and Guilleminault,

C. (1990) Maxillary, mandibular and hyoid advancement for treatment of obstructive sleep apnea: a review of 40 patients. *J. Oral Maxillofac. Surg.*, **48**, 20–6.

24. Hasan, A., McGuigan, J., Morgan, M.D.L. and Matthews, H.R. (1989) Minitracheotomy: a simple alternative to tracheostomy in obstructive sleep apnoea. *Thorax*, **44**, 224–5.

25. Eveloff, S.E., Rosenberg, C.L., Carlisle, C.C. and Millman, R.P. (1993) Determinants of efficacy of a mandibular advancement device for the treatment of OSA. *Am. Rev. Respir. Dis.*, **147**, A252.

26. Hoffstein, V., Mateika, S. and Metes, A. (1993) Effect of nasal dilation on snoring and apneas during different stages of sleep. *Sleep*, **16**, 360–5.

27. Brownell, L.G., West, P. Sweatman, P. *et al.* (1982) Protriptyline in obstructive sleep apnea. A double-blind trial. *N. Engl. J. Med.*, **307**, 1037–42.

28. Bonora, M., St John, W.M. and Bledsoe, T.A. (1985) Differential elevation by protriptyline and depression by diazepam of upper airway respiratory motor activity. *Am. Rev. Respir. Dis.*, **131**, 41–5.

29. Series, F. and Marc, I. (1993) Effects of protriptyline on snoring characteristics. *Chest*, **104**, 14–18.

30. Rajagopal, K.R., Bennett, L.L. and Dillard, T.A. (1986) Overnight nasal CPAP improves hypersomnolence in sleep apnea. *Chest*, **90**, 172–6.

31. Takasaki, Y., Orr, D., Popkin, J. *et al.* (1989) Effect of nasal continuous positive airway pressure on sleep apnea in congestive heart failure. *Am. Rev. Respir. Dis.*, **140**, 1578–84.

32. Rasanen, J., Vaisanen, I.T., Hikkila, J. and Nikki, P. (1985) Acute myocardial infarction complicated by left ventricular dysfunction and respiratory failure: the effects of continuous airway pressure. *Chest*, **87**, 158–62.

33. Brett, A. and Sinclair, D.G. (1993) Use of continuous positive airway pressure in the management of community acquired pneumonia. *Thorax*, **48**, 1280–1.

34. Wiltshire, N., Kendrick, A.H. and Catterall, J.R. (1994) Comparison of nine different nasal CPAP systems. *Thorax*, **49**, 412P.

35. Simonds, A.K., Cramer, D. and Wedzicha, J. (1991) Nasal plugs (Adams circuit) for the delivery of CPAP and non-invasive intermittent positive pressure ventilation. *Thorax*, **46**, 291P (Abstr.).

36. Engelman, H.M., Martin, S.E. and Douglas, N.J. (1994) Compliance with CPAP therapy in patients with the sleep apnoea/hypopnoea syndrome. *Thorax*, **149**, 263–6.

37. Davies, R.J.O., Vardi-Visy, K., Clarke, M. and Stradling, J.R. (1993) Identification of sleep disruption and sleep disordered breathing profile from systolic blood pressure profile. *Thorax*, **48**, 1242–7.

38. Reeves-Hoche, M.K., Hudgel, D., Meck, R. and Zwillich, C.W. (1993) BiPAP vs CPAP: patient compliance in the treatment of obstructive sleep apnea, six month data in a two year study. *Am. Rev. Respir, Dis.*, **147**, A251.

39. Elliott, M.W., Aquilina, R., Green, M. *et al.* (1994) A comparison of different modes of non-invasive ventilatory support: effects on ventilation and inspiratory muscle effort. *Anaesthesia*, **49**, 279–83.

40. Hoffstein, V., Viner, S., Mateika, S. and Conway, J. (1992) Treatment of obstructive sleep apnea with nasal continuous positive airway pressure. Patient compliance, perception of benefits, and side effects. *Am. Rev. Respir. Dis.*, **145**, 841–5.

41. Pepin, J.L., Levy, P., Leger P. *et al.* (1993) Are patients education and technical and medical follow-up able to increase compliance with therapy in chronic respiratory patients? *Eur. Respir. J.*, **6**, 380s.

42. Kribbs, N.B., Pack, A.I., Kline, L.R. and Smith, P.L. (1993) Objective measurement of patterns of nasal CPAP use by patients with obstructive sleep apnea. *Am. Rev. Respir. Dis.*, **147**, 887–95.

43. Reeves-Hoche, M.K., Meck, R. and Zwillich, C.W. (1994) Nasal CPAP: an objective evaluation of patient compliance. *Am. Rev. Respir. Dis.*, **149**, 149–54.

44. Smeets, F. (1994) Travel for technology-dependent patients with respiratory disease. *Thorax*, **49**, 77–81.

14

Physiotherapy and nasal intermittent positive pressure ventilation

JULIA BOTT and FIDELMA MORAN

INTRODUCTION: PHYSIOTHERAPY AND ITS AIMS

Physiotherapy is 'a healthcare profession which emphasizes the use of physical approaches in the prevention and treatment of disease and disability' [1]. In respiratory care, physiotherapy treatment is achieved through a combination of assessment, advice and education, and hands-on intervention.

The aims of respiratory physiotherapy are to:

- Reduce fear and anxiety.
- Reduce breathlessness and the work of breathing.
- Improve efficiency of ventilation.
- Mobilize and aid expectoration of secretions.
- Improve knowledge and understanding.
- Reduce (thoracic) pain.
- Maintain or improve exercise tolerance and functional ability.

Nasal intermittent positive pressure ventilation is both a technique designed to improve ventilation and a 'physical treatment'. There is debate as to whether physiotherapists are the most suitable health care professionals to administer NIPPV. However, in many institutions they will form a key part of the team that delivers this treatment.

Individuals who require ventilatory support have an abnormal respiratory pattern and may be breathless, anxious or confused. The health care professional in this situation needs to be patient, calm and confident with good patient handling skills. Knowledge and understanding of respiratory physiology and equipment are also essential. Respiratory physiotherapists are likely to have all the prerequisite skills, with a distinct core skill being patient handling, a vital ingredient in the success of non-invasive techniques [2] in acute respiratory failure.

The techniques of applying NIPPV are covered in other sections of this book. For the purposes of this chapter we will identify standard physiotherapy treatments, with reference to the aims that they fulfil, and explore their modifications and adaptations for the patient receiving NIPPV.

A careful assessment of a patient is 'the linchpin of physiotherapy' [3] and initially an assessment should be made at each visit. A first general premise is that physiotherapy treatment must be realistic, effective and, above all, acceptable to the patient in all but extreme circumstances.

Non-Invasive Respiratory Support. Edited by Anita Simonds. Published by Chapman & Hall, London. ISBN 0412 56840 3.

THE PATIENT'S PROBLEMS AND RELEVANT PHYSIOTHERAPY ACTION

FEAR AND ANXIETY

The reduction of a patient's fear and anxiety is an integral part of physiotherapy care. Anxiety can be greatly increased if patients do not understand their condition or the ventilatory equipment around them, or if their breathing feels 'out of control'. Good communication, counselling and health education all play their part in alleviating a patient's stress [4]. The following techniques may all be helpful.

Reassurance

Throughout the treatment of any patient, careful explanation, constant reassurance and praise are key factors, combined with relaxation techniques, if appropriate. When NIPPV is introduced electively to a patient in a relatively stable condition, e.g. patients with slowly worsening chronic respiratory failure, it can be introduced gradually over a prolonged period. This allows time to familiarize with the technique, the equipment and its care. This extra time also provides opportunity for discussion and questions that will help allay both patients' and carers' anxieties.

When a patient is admitted in an acute or critical condition, this gradual introduction to the technique is not always possible. In this situation, as the equipment is introduced, careful explanation of its function and use should be given and reiterated as frequently as necessary.

Advice and explanation

The physiotherapist, along with other members of the multidisciplinary team, will need to provide or reinforce the patient's knowledge and understanding of his or her disease, the equipment, its use and expected benefits and shortcomings. When able, the patient should be taught how to use and care for the equipment. Because NIPPV is a simple technique, most patients soon learn to handle the equipment independently. In addition, the increased ventilation and improved blood gases lead to an improvement in mental state. The patient, consequently, is thus more able to cooperate in his or her own medical management, leading to increased self-sufficiency. This is frequently very beneficial for building self-esteem [4].

Relaxation

Although the teaching of formal relaxation techniques would not be appropriate in an acutely ill patient, helping a breathless patient to relax will assist in reducing his or her anxiety level. Moreover, relaxation, combined with other techniques (see below) may help reduce the work of breathing and will improve synchronization of respiration with the ventilator.

BREATHLESSNESS, INCREASED WORK OF BREATHING, AND INEFFICIENT VENTILATION

Physiotherapy has much to offer the patient who is breathless. Worthwhile improvement can be achieved by apparently simple measures.

Positioning

The positioning of patients for comfort, for the reduction of the work of breathing and for the optimization of the ventilation/perfusion ratio is commonly the first step in any physiotherapy treatment. The right position will help alleviate breathlessness and will vary depending on the individual and underlying pathology. High sitting,

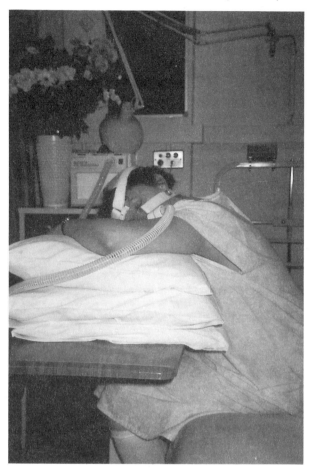

Fig. 14.1 Forward lean sitting (FLS) position.

forward lean sitting (FLS) (Fig. 14.1) and high side-lying are comfortable positions, provided the patient is well supported. All patients ventilated with NIPPV should be encouraged to adopt a comfortable and relaxed posture.

In severely breathless patients with hyper-inflated lungs and low, flat diaphragms the FLS position may be used for the delivery of NIPPV. The key features of this position are that the patient should be comfortable, with the arms, and thus the shoulder girdle, fully supported on a table with appropriate num-

bers of pillows to support the head and allow the patient to relax. The position may be adopted in a chair or sitting over the edge of the bed. Caution needs to be exercised in the patient with severe ankle oedema, with appropriate modifications to the position to minimize further swelling.

In patients with severe chronic obstructive pulmonary disease (COPD), FLS has been shown to bring about a decrease in the work of breathing [5], a reduction in the sensation of breathlessness [5,6,7] and a decrease in expiratory reserve volume and minute ventilation, without detriment to arterial blood gas tensions [7]. These benefits may be due to the improvement in the length:tension ratio of the diaphragm in this position [5,6].

Breathing control

In conjunction with positioning, breathing control should be taught on and off the ventilator. Breathing control is 'gentle breathing using the lower chest with relaxation of the upper chest and shoulders. It is breathing at normal tidal volume and at a natural rate. Expiration is unforced' [8]. Optimal ventilation with NIPPV attempts to mimic breathing control and patients should be encouraged to relax during ventilation. The aim should be for the patient to utilize breathing control in everyday life and, in particular, when breathless or during activity.

IPPB and CPAP

If the simpler techniques provide insufficient relief or effect, intermittent positive pressure breathing (IPPB) or continuous positive airway pressure (CPAP) can be used. Non-invasive patient-triggered ventilation in the form of IPPB [8] has been used by chest physiotherapists for many years [9]. IPPB has been shown to increase ventilation [10,11] and reduce the work of breathing when the patient is synchronized with the machine [12,13]. CPAP increases functional residual capacity and reduces the work of breathing in proportion to the level of pressure delivered [14]. Studies have shown that NIPPV also reduces the work of breathing, and may be more effective than CPAP in this respect [15]. Moreover, patients with an acute exacerbation of COPD receiving NIPPV are less breathless than controls [16]. Therefore, for patients on NIPPV, the use of IPPB or CPAP for this purpose is usually superfluous.

In some patients, however, IPPB may be more comfortable or more effective than NIPPV in increasing basal expansion for chest clearance. If this is the case, the two forms of ventilation can be alternated as necessary.

SECRETIONS

In the authors' clinical experience, especially of COPD patients, spontaneous clearance of secretions is usually possible once the patient is adequately ventilated with NIPPV. Should the removal of secretions be a problem, any, or all, of the following techniques may need to be employed. Depending on the underlying diagnosis, bronchodilator therapy may need to be given prior to chest clearance treatments (see below).

Humidification

Patients receiving NIPPV may well be dehydrated, causing further impairment of mucociliary clearance. The patient should, therefore, be encouraged to take fluids, if allowed. If the patient is well orientated and motivated, drinking during NIPPV can be taught. The patient is instructed to sip small amounts carefully through a straw, swallowing on expiration. Not all patients can achieve the cordination required and drinking is contraindicated in confused subjects. Eating while on NIPPV should *not* be allowed. Maintenance humidification can be achieved by a heat and moisture exchanger in the circuit. For added humidification a heated water bath device is suitable (see Fig. 10.1). A degree of humidification can be achieved with saline nebulizers, given as frequently as the patient requires.

The active cycle of breathing techniques

An example of the active cycle of breathing techniques (ACBT) is a series of techniques performed in the sequence outlined below:

136

- Breathing control.
- 3/4 thoracic expansion exercises.
- Breathing control.
- 3/4 thoracic expansion exercises.
- Breathing control.
- Forced expiration technique.
- Breathing control.

The key features are to allow the patient plenty of time for relaxation and recovery and to avoid extreme effort. A detailed description of the technique is found in Webber and Pryor [8]. ACBT has been demonstrated to be an effective method of aiding the removal of secretions [17], with no detriment to arterial oxygen saturation [18] and some improvement in pulmonary function [19].

The equivalent of breathing control is achieved by using the normal settings on the ventilator. Increased expansion (equivalent to thoracic expansion exercises) is achieved by increasing tidal volume (or pressure, if a pressure cycled machine is used). For planned huffing combined with breathing control

(the forced expiration technique, FET), or coughing, the tubing at the expiratory valve should be disconnected. This prevents the patient having to work against inspiratory pressure from the ventilator. The ACBT can be performed in forward lean sitting, supported sitting, high side-lying and in postural drainage or modified postural drainage positions.

Chest clapping and shaking/vibrations

These remain controversial techniques. However, there is some evidence that, in patients with copious secretions, chest clapping is an effective addition to ACBT [20] (Fig. 14.2). If chest clapping is added during NIPPV, it should be carried out during periods of increased tidal volume. Chest shaking or vibrations can be performed during the expiratory phase, as with spontaneous respiration, but bearing in mind that the expiratory phase is shortened, and that such forced manoeuvres are strongly contraindicated during inspiration.

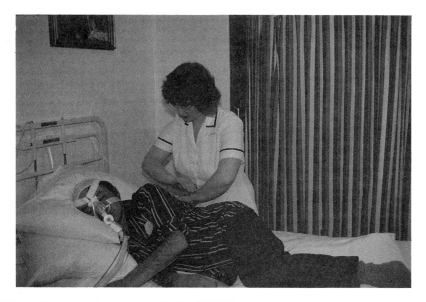

Fig. 14.2 Aiding clearance of secretions during NIPPV.

Postural drainage

In patients who are spontaneously breathing, gravity assisted, postural drainage (PD) positions may increase clearance of excess bronchial secretions [21]. For the patient unable to tolerate full PD positions, modified positions can be adopted, e.g. alternate side-lying. For some patients, PD may only be possible with the assisted ventilatory support of NIPPV or IPPB.

Intermittent positive pressure breathing

IPPB is a technique used by physiotherapists for patients who are not self-ventilating adequately or who are too confused, weak or exhausted to clear secretions effectively [9].

We have found it of clinical value to use IPPB periodically in place of NIPPV if it provides:

- more effective expansion;
- better coordination for chest shaking/ vibrations;
- relief of facial pressure areas/ claustrophobia;
- more effective administration of bronchodilators;
- greater subjective or objective benefit to the patient.

Suctioning

In extreme instances, naso- or oropharyngeal suctioning may be needed, with or without an artificial airway inserted. In this situation the patient will often be drowsy, have sputum retention and, despite the physiotherapist's best efforts to induce a spontaneous cough, will be unable to cough effectively. All the standard precautions should be adhered to [2] and the NIPPV mask will need to be temporarily, and as briefly as possible, removed. It is imperative that the patient is adequately oxygenated throughout this procedure.

When a patient in the terminal stages of disease is distressed by secretions in the upper airways, only oropharyngeal suction with the Yankauer sucker may be appropriate. Alternatively, preparations to dry the secretions may be preferred, e.g. hyoscine hydrobromide.

Other techniques

Alternative treatments which may be used for chest clearance include autogenic drainage [22], positive expiratory pressure (PEP) mask [23] and the Flutter VRP1 (VarioRaw) [8]. The effectiveness of these techniques combined with NIPPV has not been assessed, but they are unlikely to be of additional benefit [24]. However, any patient who has experienced subjective benefit, or who wishes to try a particular treatment, should be informed of all the advantages and drawbacks and then given the opportunity to choose his or her own preferred treatment [25].

THORACIC PAIN

Physiotherapists are skilled at the assessment and treatment of pain. Various modalities may be employed, e.g. heat, manual therapies, acupuncture, interferential, transcutaneous electrical nerve stimulation (TENS). Description and discussion of these techniques is beyond the scope of this chapter. However, many such techniques may be successfully employed in patients receiving NIPPV.

REDUCED EXERCISE TOLERANCE AND FUNCTIONAL ABILITY

Individual exercise programmes should be tailored to the severity of patients' disease and their ability. Training should be discontinued in the acutely ill [26]. It is possible to mobilize a patient (e.g. bed to chair) or even perform more formal exercise while on

NIPPV. Ventilator settings may need to be altered to accommodate the increased need for ventilation. Reassurance is particularly helpful during exercise sessions. Functional activities of daily living should be encouraged as soon as the patient is able. This will promote and maintain self-efficacy, either on or off the ventilator.

THE OVERALL APPROACH

It is essential that the patient receiving NIPPV is viewed holistically by the multidisciplinary team so that aspects of nutrition, occupational therapy and nursing care are not overlooked.

NUTRITIONAL SUPPORT

Eating is contraindicated while receiving NIPPV, due to the risk of aspiration under positive pressure. Some patients on NIPPV require an individualized diet. If the patient is to be fed nasogastrically, liaison with the dietician is important, as the smallest bore tube acceptable must be used, to minimize leak around the mask. Drinking, if allowed, should be encouraged, as should the intake of prescribed supplements between treatments, as directed by the dietician. Carbonated drinks and charcoal biscuits can help relieve abdominal distension caused by swallowing air. Physiotherapy treatments should be performed, if possible, before meals, to avoid the risk of nausea or vomiting or subsequent loss of appetite.

TERMINAL CARE

For the terminally ill patient for whom physiotherapy has been an integral part of daily life, treatment should not suddenly be withdrawn. Treatment here is aimed at keeping the patient comfortable, with particular emphasis on positioning, reassur-ance and assistance with the removal of distressing secretions. Other interventions any be added if requested. The health care professionals must bear in mind that the patient may have seen friends or fellow patients in a similar situation, the outcome being only one of transplantation, improvement or death.

As the patient's condition deteriorates synchronization with the machine becomes more difficult, despite alterations of settings. The physiotherapist needs to be sensitive to the fact that patients and relatives may 'blame' the equipment for not working. When and whether the machine should be disconnected or removed and replaced by a simple oxygen mask is dependent on each individual case. The wishes of the patient and the relatives should be considered by the multidisciplinary team. This also applies to the decision to disconnect alarms. The patient's dignity must be preserved at all times.

PRACTICAL CONSIDERATIONS

Pressure area care

In association with the nursing staff, physiotherapists need to be aware of good general skin care and encourage appropriate mobilization of the patient to prevent skin breakdown. In addition, for the patient on NIPPV, the bridge of the nose and the upper lip area are susceptible to pressure exerted by the nasal mask (see Chapter 5). Caution needs to be exercised in the prolonged wearing of a nasal mask, however comfortable, because of the risks of skin trauma. Regular checking, as with any pressure area, is essential. For some patients the mask is made more comfortable by lining it with self-adhesive towelling (such as is used for binding racquet handles), applied over a layer of cling-film wrap.

Bronchodilator therapy

For the most part, bronchodilators may easily be administered by the prescribed method when the patient is not using the ventilator. For patients unable to discontinue NIPPV for even brief periods, bronchodilator therapy can be administered concurrently via a mouthpiece run off a compressor (Fig. 14.3). Patients may find it difficult to co-ordinate inspiration through the mouthpiece with NIPPV, but often claim subjective improvement.

Oxygen

Supplemental oxygen, entrained via the porthole, should be increased prior to active physiotherapy, or added if necessary. Although the inspired oxygen concentration is not known, the physiotherapist can either use a pulse oximeter to ensure the patient is adequately oxygenated during treatment, or agree with the medical staff an appropriate amount to entrain, or both.

In addition, the physiotherapist may need to consider the oxygen outlet requirement for the patient on NIPPV, which are:

- Venturi mask;
- entrainment through port in nasal mask;
- (IPPB).

Electrical supply

Electrical points may be required for the following equipment:

- ventilator equipment;
- humidification equipment;
- compressor;
- intravenous pumps;
- (light).

All electrical and oxygen leads should be clearly marked in case of emergency.

Mask/mouth leak

The careful selection of the right size mask will pay dividends in the long run and a

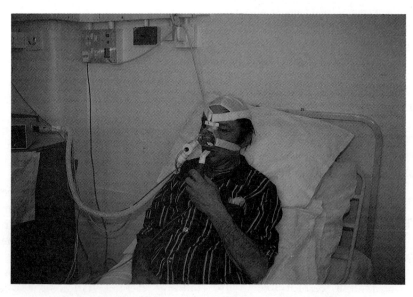

Fig. 14.3 Delivery of nebulized bronchodilator via mouthpiece during NIPPV.

correctly fitting mask may be sufficient to avoid mask leak. The mask should not simply be tightened if leak is a problem, as this puts the pressure areas at risk. Rather, the mask should be loosened, or removed, and reapplied. The cushions should be opened as wide as possible and the mask pulled downwards over the nose, before strapping into place. Towelling can be effective in some patients when applied as for pressure area care (Fig. 14.4). The correction of leaks is covered in Chapter 5.

Adverse clinical signs

At any time during the assessment and treatment of a patient on NIPPV, the physiotherapist should seek medical assistance if there is unexplained, sudden or prolonged:

- increased patient distress;
- increased airway pressure;

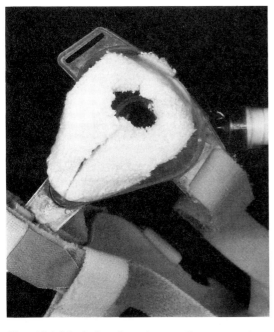

Fig. 14.4 Mask lined with towelling to reduce leaks.

- decreased oxygen saturation;
- decreased synchronization with the ventilator;
- abnormal chest wall movement.

The possibility of pneumothorax will need to be eliminated if these clinical signs do not reveal sputum plugging or any other readily identifiable cause.

CONCLUSION

Patients using NIPPV require a team approach. The physiotherapist's involvement in the management of the ventilator for the patient on NIPPV will depend on local conditions. At yet, there is still much debate on this potential role. As a profession, important issues other than merely who is *able* to facilitate this treatment, such as whether or not it is feasible to provide the manpower and the necessary 24 hour cover, need to be addressed [2].

Regardless of local arrangements regarding the ventilator, the physiotherapist has a crucial role to play with respect to psychological support, relief of pain and breathlessness, sputum clearance, exercise tolerance and functional activity.

ACKNOWLEDGEMENTS

We wish to thank Barbara A. Webber and Jennifer A. Pryor for their helpful and constructive comments and Nikki Potter for her practical help with the photography. We are grateful to the staff of the Mater Misericordiae Hospital, Dublin, and the physiotherapy staff of the London Chest Hospital for their support; in particular, Christine Mikelsons.

REFERENCES

1. Chartered Society of Physiotherapy (1991) *Curriculum of study*, pp. 12–13.
2. Bott, J., Keilty, S.E.J., Brown, A.M. and Ward, E.M. (1992) Nasal intermittent positive

pressure ventilation. *Physiotherapy*, **78**, 93–6.

3. Hough, A. (1991) *Physiotherapy in Respiratory Care. A Problem-Solving Approach.* Chapman & Hall, London.

4. Sim, J. (1993) Communication, counselling and health education, in *Physiotherapy for Respiratory and Cardiac Problems* (eds B.A. Webber and J.A. Pryor), Churchill Livingstone, Edinburgh, pp. 173–86.

5. O'Neill, S. and McCarthy, D.S. (1983) Postural relief of dyspnoea in severe chronic airflow limitation. *Thorax*, **38**, 595–600.

6. Sharp, J.T., Drutz, W.S., Moisan, T. *et al.* (1980) Postural relief of dyspnea in severe chronic obstructive pulmonary disease. *Am. Rev. Respir. Dis.*, **122**, 201–11.

7. Barach, A.L. (1974) Chronic lung disease: postural relief of dyspnea. *Arch. Phys. Med. Rehabil.*, **55**, 494–504.

8. Webber, B.A. and Pryor, J.A. (1993) Physiotherapy skills: techniques and adjuncts, in *Physiotherapy for Respiratory and Cardiac Problems* (eds B.A. Webber and J.A. Pryor), Churchill Livingstone, Edinburgh, pp. 113–71.

9. Bott, J., Keilty, S.E.J. and Noone, L. (1992) Intermittent positive pressure breathing – A dying art? *Physiotherapy*, **78**, 656–60.

10. Emmanuel, G.E., Smith, W.M. and Brisco, W.A. (1966) The effect of IPPB and voluntary hyper-ventilation upon the distribution of ventilation and pulmonary blood flow to the lung in COPD. *J. Clin. Invest.*, **45**, 1221–32.

11. Torres, G., Lyons, H.A. and Emerson, P. (1960) The effects of IPPB on the interpulmonary distribution of inspired air. *Am. J. Med.*, **29**, 946.

12. Sukumalchantra, Y., Park, S.S. and Williams, M.H. (1965) The effect of intermittent positive pressure breathing (IPPB) in acute ventilatory failure. *Am. Rev. Respir. Dis.*, **92**, 885.

13. Ayres, S.M., Kozam, R.L. and Lukas, D.S. (1963) The effects of intermittent positive pressure breathing on intrathoracic pressure, pulmonary mechanics and the work of breathing. *Am. Rev. Respir. Dis.*, **87**, 370–9.

14. Gherini, S., Peters, R.M. and Virgilio, R.W. (1979) Mechanical work of breathing with positive end expiratory pressure and continuous positive airways pressure. *Chest*, **76**, 251–6.

15. Elliott, M.W., Aquilina, R., Green, M. *et al.* (1994) A comparison of different modes of non-invasive ventilatory support: effects on ventilation and inspiratory muscle effort. *Anaesthesia*, **49**, 270–83.

16. Bott, J., Carroll, M.P., Conway, J.H. *et al.* (1993) Randomised controlled trial of nasal ventilation in acute ventilatory failure due to chronic obstructive airways disease. *Lancet*, **341**, 1555–7.

17. Pryor, J.A., Webber, B.A., Hodson, M.E. and Batten, J.C. (1979) Evaluation of the forced expiration technique as an adjunct to postural drainage in the treatment of cystic fibrosis. *Br. Med. J.*, **2**, 417–18.

18. Pryor, J.A., Webber, B.A. and Hodson, M.E., (1990) Effect of chest physiotherapy on oxygen saturation in patients with cystic fibrosis. *Thorax*, **45**, 77.

19. Webber, B.A., Hofmeyr, J.L., Morgan, M.D.L. and Hodson, M.E. (1986) Effects of postural drainage, incorporating the forced expiration technique, on pulmonary function in cystic fibrosis. *Br. J. Dis. Chest*, **80**, 353–9.

20. Gallon, A. (1991) Evaluation of chest percussion in the treatment of patients with copious sputum production. *Respir. Med.*, **85**, 45–51.

21. Sutton, P.P., Parker, R.A., Webber, B.A. *et al.* (1983) Assessment of the forced expiration technique, postural drainage and directed coughing in chest physiotherapy. *Eur. J. Respir. Dis.*, **64**, 62–8.

22. David, A. (1993) Autogenic drainage – the German approach, in *Respiratory Care* (ed. J.A. Pryor), Churchill Livingstone, Edinburgh, pp. 65–78.

23. Falk, M. and Andersen, J.B. (1991) Positive expiratory pressure (PEP) mask, in *Respiratory Care* (ed. J.A. Pryor), Churchill Livingstone, Edinburgh, pp. 51–64.

24. Pryor, J.A. (1991) The forced expiration technique, in *Respiratory Care* (ed. J.A. Pryor), Churchill Livingstone, Edinburgh, pp. 79–98.

25. Latimer, T. (1991) Caring for seriously ill and dying patients: the philosophy and physics. *Canad. Med. Assoc. J.*, **1**, 859–64.

26. Dodd, M.E. (1991) Exercise in cystic fibrosis adults, in *Respiratory Care* (ed. J.A. Pryor), Churchill Livingstone, Edinburgh, pp. 27–50.

15

The home ventilatory care network

ANITA K. SIMONDS

INTRODUCTION

The transfer of care from hospital to home needs to be achieved as seamlessly as possible. It has been suggested [1] that the goals of long-term home ventilation should be:

- to extend life;
- to enhance the quality of life;
- to reduce morbidity;
- to improve physical and physiological function;
- to deliver treatment cost-effectively.

It is self-evident that patients should be medically stable at the time of discharge, with no imminent change predicted in their clinical state or ventilatory needs. Motivation of the patient and his or her family is hugely important. No discharge will work unless the recipient is committed to ventilatory support and believes it will benefit him/her.

HOME CARE NETWORK

The success of any home care programme depends on a support network which inspires confidence in all parties. Such a network has several components.

1. (a) Ready access to medical advice, home visits, hospital admission and respite care.
   (b) Regular monitoring of medical progress.
2. Technical support:
   (a) replacment of disposables and hardware;
   (b) emergency equipment breakdown repair service;
   (c) regular maintenance of equipment in the patient's home.
3. Patient and family education. Training of caregivers.
4. Close liaison with the general practitioner and other medical and ancillary teams involved with care.
5. Advice regarding holidays, transportation of equipment, fitness for airline travel, social service entitlements.
6. Patient support schemes (International Ventilator Users Network, Breathe Easy clubs, Muscular Dystrophy Association, Motor Neurone Disease Association, Scoliosis Association UK, Brompton Breathers etc.).

No individual should be discharged without a support network in place, although the level of back-up support required will vary from patient to patient.

Non-Invasive Respiratory Support. Edited by Anita Simonds. Published by Chapman & Hall, London. ISBN 0412 56840 3.

ACCESS TO MEDICAL ADVICE

Patients and their families will inevitably need medical guidance from time to time, e.g. whether to start a course of antibiotics, queries about ventilator settings, or the side-effects of treatment such as nasal bridge sores and gastric distension. These may be simply dealt with by telephone, or require a home visit, outpatient assessment or admission. A team member with adequate experience of ventilatory support should be available on a 24 hour basis to triage the calls and arrange suitable follow-up. *All* patients should have access to a telephone. Individuals should be able to self-refer for admission if their condition rapidly deteriorates. Other hospital departments such as the Accident and Emergency Unit should be aware of these procedures. An open access 'walk-in' clinic for patients receiving non-invasive ventilation and CPAP, staffed by a respiratory support technician/nurse is very helpful for sorting out minor technical difficulties, before they develop into major problems. During home visits the clinical state of the patient and ventilator performance can be assessed. A portable oximeter and vitalograph are useful for these visits. The frequency of routine follow-up assessments will vary from patient to patient. Shared care is particularly helpful for patients who live long distances from the ventilation centre and often serves as a stimulus for the development of local home ventilation programmes.

TECHNICAL SUPPORT

Patients need to have an action plan to put into practice if their ventilatory equipment malfunctions. Many using nocturnal non-invasive ventilation will cope for several days without ventilatory support; highly ventilator-dependent patients will need an immediate solution to the mechanical problem. For patients who cannot breathe independently for more than a few hours a 'back-up' ventilator is essential. Similarly a battery option should be available to cope with power cuts and travel outside the home. (The electrical authority can be notified in the UK so that power reconnection after a power cut will occur as a priority in ventilator users.)

In the UK there are several nationwide service and maintenance schemes which are coordinated by the large hospital units and carried out by engineers from the commercial sector. Patients from other hospitals can be entered in these schemes. It is helpful to categorize patients as to their degree of ventilatory dependency. This allows engineers to give precedence to those who require urgent attention. A simple way to do this is on the basis of one night, two night and three night need, i.e. a 'one night' patient cannot function for more than one disturbed night without a ventilator, a 'two night' patient cannot cope for more than two nights etc. Patients are asked to notify the equipment problem by telephone to the coordinating centre. This call should be screened to ensure that there is no simple remedy to the problem (e.g. change of fuse). The engineer is then contacted. Ideally, the technical problem is dealt with in the patient's home, but if a repair cannot be effected a substitute ventilator of the same make is provided. An alternative is for service and maintenance to be carried out by the local hospital. This may work well, but it should be remembered that ventilators can break down at weekends and on public holidays when many in-hospital biomedical engineering departments are closed. Patients often have great difficulty in transporting their equipment to the hospital.

Finally, some manufacturers and dealers offer service and maintenance deals for their own brand of ventilator or CPAP machine. Not all of these schemes include a 24-hour breakdown service and so would be inappropriate in a highly ventilator-dependent individual.

Home ventilators need servicing once or twice a year depending on the model. This will include a check on electrical safety. CPAP machines should be serviced once a year. Oxygen concentrators are independently serviced by the providing company, e.g. Devilbiss.

Disposables such as masks, headgear, tubing etc. can be supplied by the hospital or direct from the manufacturers. On average recipients of mask ventilation will need one to two commercial masks a year. Customized facepieces have a variable lifespan. New ventilator tubing and headgear is needed once a year. Occasional patients benefit from a disposable heat and moisture exchanger (e.g. Portex thermovent) when secretions or rhinitis are a problem. These should be discarded after 24–48 hours.

Tracheostomy-IPPV patients have a far greater requirement for technical support in the home [2] and a full description of their needs is beyond the scope of this text. However, support equipment should include suction machine and suction tubes, spare tracheostomy tube, stoma dressings, gloves, saline, syringes and humidifier.

PATIENT AND FAMILY EDUCATION

All ventilator users, and their families and carers, need to understand the nature of their underlying respiratory condition, its consequences and, where possible, the overall prognosis. They also need to understand the basic principles of the ventilator and be provided with a simple problem-solving approach to medical or technical problems in the home. Before discharge the patient/main carer should be able to demonstrate that he/she can connect the ventilator, mask and tubing correctly and that they understand the function of the alarms. It is helpful to provide a patient-orientated handbook on these pratical aspects which should include a clear state-

ment of the patient's ventilatory settings, and oxgen flow rate if applicable.

Patients are also responsible for the routine maintenance of their ventilatory equipment, which will include changing or washing the filters on positive pressure ventilators, and rinsing the mask and tubing. The mask and ventilator tubing should be washed in soapy water every week and dried thoroughly. Sterilization is not required and may damage the mask. Individuals using negative pressure equipment will need to wash pneumojackets regularly.

The training of patients and carers regarding T-IPPV is necessarily more detailed. Carers need to be competent in suction and changing or replacing the tracheostomy tube.

Ideally, for the patient and carer home ventilation should form part of a comprehensive pulmonary/neuromuscular rehabilitation programme.

LIAISON WITH OTHER TEAM MEMBERS

Clear information on the patient's medical and ventilatory requirements needs to be available to all involved parties, and they should be involved in decision-making at every opportunity. It is helpful for other team members to have a copy of the ventilator handbook.

ADVICE REGARDING TRAVELLING WITH THE VENTILATOR/BENEFITS

As indicated in Chapter 8, many patients receiving nocturnal non-invasive ventilation return to a near normal quality of life and understandably want to take part in normal activities, including foreign travel. This is usually feasible in nocturnal non-invasive ventilator users and, with planning, more handicapped individuals with well-controlled respiratory failure can also travel extensively. NIPPV ventilators are easier to transport than portable nPV systems, which tend to be bulky. Independent arrangements regarding oxygen requirements and transportation of ventilatory equipment should be made well in advance. The fitness of any individual to fly depends on their general health, baseline Pa_{O_2} and Pa_{CO_2}, ventilatory dependency, the altitude (cabin pressurization), duration of flight and level of physical activity during the flight. Uncontrolled hypercapnia, severe hypercapnia in response to oxygen therapy and bullous lung disease are all contraindications to air travel. 'Fitness to fly' tests where the arterial blood gas tensions are measured before and during a simulated flight are very helpful for calculating oxygen requirements and ensuring that hypercapnia is not precipitated. As ventilation will inevitably deteriorate during sleep in those who require nocturnal ventilatory support and obstructive sleep apnoea will become manifest without CPAP, patients are advised not to sleep during the flight. Short-haul fights or stop-overs are therefore preferable to long-haul flights. The ventilator should travel as cabin luggage. Patients should be provided with a letter from their medical attendant to authorize this requirement. The BiPAP (Respironics) machine is dual voltage and useful for trips to North America. The standard voltage in other destinations should be checked and a suitable plug obtained.

A Eurolung Assistance scheme has been set up for ventilator- and oxygen-dependent travellers [3]. This is an association of health professionals, medical technology services, tourism agencies and insurance companies which promotes travel in such patients. The Eurolung Assistance Directory published by the group provides useful information on the availability of support services, including oxygen suppliers throughout Europe, and also gives details of specific airline requirements for technology-dependent individuals (see Appendix B for address).

SUPPORT GROUPS

Many patients and families find it valuable to share their experiences. Addresses of relevant agencies are given in Appendix B. Some hospitals provide newsletters and research undates on ventilatory equipment.

The transfer of medical high technology to the community has gained momentum over the past decade. Home ventilation has played a pioneering role in developing high and medium technology care in the home as domiciliary support was first introduced during the poliomyelitis epidemics 50 years ago. The most significant recent changes have been the widening of indications for home respiratory support, the introduction of improved ventilatory methods and monitoring equipment, and the realization that patients with ventilatory failure due to a variety of causes may be returned to near normal function by using ventilatory assistance soley during sleep. Although the number of recipients of T-IPPV has increased, the greatest expansion has been in patients using non-invasive ventilation, particularly nasal ventilation at night. This has important cost implications as the level of care and general home support needed for T-IPPV patients clearly exceeds that of individuals using non-invasive ventilation, may of whom are fully employed.

WORLD PERSPECTIVE

It has been estimated that 8000 people worldwide receive long-term mechanical ventilation in the home for more than a few hours a day [4]. This compares to around 5000 individuals in the USA alone treated with domiciliary oxygen therapy.

The organization of home care has evolved very differently in the UK, the rest of Europe and the USA. Provision of respiratory support remains rudimentary in many countries.

France has a well-developed home respiratory care system which may serve as a useful role model. The French system of home respiratory care and other programmes throughout Europe are discussed in detail in the following chapter, where home ventilation will be set in the context of other respiratory therapies in the home (LTOT and CPAP). Here, the organization of home ventilation in the USA and UK is contrasted.

THE USA

Home ventilation has a long track record in the USA, with around 5000 patients receiving home ventilatory support. American guidelines [1] and a consensus document [5] have been published on the provision of treatment. These have established criteria for the evaluation of suitable candidates, and examined discharge policy, ventilatory principles unique to children and acceptable levels of home care. Despite these efforts, there is no national policy, administrative structure or system for funding long-term ventilation. As a result, not all patients who warrant home ventilation receive it, and in others there are long delays before discharge can be arranged. Payment or reimbursement for equipment comes from a variety of sources – federal or state government, private insurance or the patient's own funds. There is no centralized data collection on ventilator use, but this situation may be corrected by initiatives such as the creation of the National Center for Mechanical Ventilation in Denver which has a responsibility for collecting information on the performance and safety of home ventilatory apparatus.

Regional information does exist, however. A survey of long-term respiratory support in Minnesota [2] has shown that the number of ventilator-assisted individuals more than doubled between 1986 and 1992. Large increases were seen in the paediatric group and in those over the age of 60 years. The most prevalent primary diagnosis was poliomyelitis, but the number in this group was relatively static compared to a marked growth in patients with cervical trauma, motor neurone disease and muscular dystrophy. No breakdown is given as to the mode of ventilatory support. However, more patients in the USA are Grade 4 ventilator-dependent (requiring 24 hour support) than in the UK.

For the Minnesota group as a whole, the average monthly cost of ventilatory support was \$6500 per patient in the home, and \$19 351 in a long-stay institution. The projected intensive care bed cost was \$64 513 per month. It is difficult to know whether this information is represenatative of activity in the USA as a whole. However, in another study, Goldberg [6] describes an initial cost reduction of 70% in a paediatric ventilatory homecare programme.

A new growth area is the use of bi-level pressure support ventilation (BiPAP, Respironics). This is a consequence of the growth in sleep laboratories which have identified an increasing number of individuals with nocturnal hypoventilation secondary to neuromuscular disease, COPD and obstructive sleep apnoea. The relative simplicity of the BiPAP equipment has led to programmes of respiratory support in institutions which previously were unable to offer this treatment. There is little information on the number of patients receiving BiPAP therapy and it is apparent that there is the potential for an explosion of unregulated use of this new treatment modality.

It remains to be seen whether US health care reforms will make cost-effective home ventilation accessible to all.

THE UNITED KINGDOM

Whereas long-term oxygen therapy is available on the National Health Service and funded centrally, there is as yet no coordinated provision of home ventilation. The Responaut˙ programme at St Thomas's Hospital, London, set up in 1965, was the earliest large-scale treatment initiative [7]. Subsequently, in the early 1980s, two other major centres, the Royal Brompton Hospital, London, and Papworth Hospital (previously Newmarket Hospital), Cambridge, began to treat patients, primarily with restrictive disorders, with negative pressure ventilation. The advent of nasal positive pressure ventilation in the mid 1980s led to a rapid expansion in patient numbers, and the introduction of home respiratory support programmes in other centres in the UK. However, these are not well distributed geographically and some regions have poor access to home ventilatory facilities. It is likely that between 800 and 1000 adults and children are currently receiving home ventilation in the UK.

Department of Health guidelines exist for the prescription of LTOT by general practitioners, generally on the advice of pulmonary physicians (see Table 7.2). There are no guidelines for home ventilation or CPAP therapy. With the purchaser-provider system of health delivery, reimbursement for hospital care, equipment costs and the manitenance of equipment in the patient's home is sought from the referring health authority. It is crucial that purchasers (usually health authorities) recognize the advantages and cost savings offered by home ventilation. Some providers are able to bulk-buy ventilators and offer a low cost lease scheme, which saves the purchaser excessive start-up costs. These schemes have the advantage that equipment can be substituted if it no longer suits the patient's ventilatory needs, or more advanced models become available. As indicated in Chapter 3, the cost of a nasal ventilator varies between £2500 and £6000. Lease schemes which offer a range of ventilators and full service and maintenance of the equipment in the recipient's home cost between £2000 and £3000 per annum.

The majority of the above deals with patients receiving non-invasive ventilation. The number of T-IPPV patients in the UK is probably less than 100. Some of these are managed by the Spinal Injuries Centre at Southport, Merseyside, which has special expertise in the management of cervical lesions. Other individuals are managed by local chest physicians, paediatricians, anaesthetists or other spinal units.

A UK home ventilator register has recently been set up under the auspices of the British Thoracic Society and may be extended to CPAP use. It is hoped that the data collected will help improve the provision of ventilatory facilities in the UK.

CPAP treatment remains a particular problem in England and Wales, where at present there is limited support from health authorities to purchase CPAP machines. Inevitably as a consequence patients who would benefit from CPAP are not receiving this, or are purchasing their own machines. However, the situation may be improving. Most insurtherapy for obstructive sleep apnoea, although a number will now support the investigation of the patient with a sleep study.

REFERENCES

1. Report of the Ad Hoc Committee, Respiratory Care Section, American College of Chest Physicians (1986) Long term mechanical ventilation. Guidelines for management in the home and at alternate community sites. *Chest*, **90**, 1S–37S.
2. Adams, A.B., Whitman, J. and Marcy, T. (1993) Survey of long-term ventilatory support in Minnesota: 1986 and 1992. *Chest*, **103**, 463–9.
3. Smeets, F. (1994) Travel for technology-dependent patients with respiratory disease. *Thorax*, **49**, 77–81.
4. Pierson, D.J. (1989) Home respiratory care in different countries. *Eur. Respir. J.*, **2**, 630s–636s.

5. Plummer, A.L., O'Donohue, W.J. and Petty, T.L. (1989) Consensus conference on problems in home mechanical ventilation. *Am. Rev. Respir. Dis.*, **140**, 555–60.

6. Goldberg, A.I., Faure, E.A.M., Vaughn, C.J. *et al.* (1984) Home care for life-supported persons: an approach to programme development. *J. Pediatr.*, **104**, 785–95.

7. Goldberg, A.I. and Faure, A.M. (1984) Home care for life-supported persons in England. The Responaut program. *Chest*, **6**, 910–14.

16

Organization of home respiratory care in Europe

PATRICK LEGER

INTRODUCTION

As was the case in the USA and the United Kingdom, the development of home respiratory care (HRC) in France resulted from the home care programmes of the poliomyelitis centres. The first home care efforts were regional, created by pioneers in the field of HRC with the financial support of the national health care system. One of the first non-profit organizations was created in Lyons in 1959, and has continued to provide support for individuals with chronic respiratory insufficiency (CRI). Since the end of the polio epidemic, HRC has grown continuously and improvements in survival rate and quality of life in selected patients using long-term HRC are incontestable [1–5].

The purpose of this chapter is to describe the organization and distribution of HRC for patients with CRI and sleep apnoea syndrome. The discussion will be limited to mechanical therapy, including LTOT, CPAP and home mechanical ventilation (HMV), but will exclude medical treatment, inhalation therapy and chest physiotherapy. By definition, HRC services are provided to individuals living at home, which is considered to be wherever the patient has permanent residence. This includes some home substitutes such as retirement homes. Discussion will be mainly focused on the French system because it is the one with which the author is most familiar, but also because it is one of the oldest systems, with a large amount of information available on patients treated over the past 30 years.

The French system of home care, its costs and reimbursement will be compared with other countries, mainly in Europe.

THE FRENCH SYSTEM

In France, two systems are available for patients needing HRC: the public non-profit association, which has been in existence for 30 years, and the private system, which has been developed significantly over the past 10 years, largely through the promotion of liquid O_2 for LTOT. Physicians are free to choose between the public or private system for HRC. The public system has responsiblity for 70% of approximately 40 000 patients treated in HRC programmes in France and will, therefore, be described in more detail [6].

The French system originated with only a few regional organizations which, as previously indicated, were created to support technology-dependent polio survivors. The system expanded at a relatively slow pace

Non-Invasive Respiratory Support. Edited by Anita Simonds. Published by Chapman & Hall, London. ISBN 0412 56840 3.

with the addition of private local pharmacies which supplied some equipment and oxygen. With the increasing realization in the 1970s of the importance of supplemental oxygen for chronic obstructive pulmonary diseases (COPD) and the technical development of oxygen concentrators, the public HRC organizations quickly multiplied and it was evident that central organization was needed. The result was the creation of a National Home Care Association for Chronic Respiratory Insufficiency (ANTADIR).

THE ROLE OF ANTADIR [7]

ANTADIR was created in 1981 to unify and organize the network of 16 existing regional oranizations. At this time the goals of ANTADIR were:

1. to complete and coordinate the national network of regional associations in order to organize the management of LTOT among them;
2. to install a purchase organization for the main equipment (O_2 concentrators, ventilators);
3. to improve the associate system towards the distribution of health care and social assistance.

At present there are 33 regional associations in France which are each responsible for between 140 and 2500 patients.

The current goals of ANTADIR include the following:

1. National negotiation for buying equipement at lower prices
2. Medical and technological coordination of the regional associations to obtain better homogeneity
3. Creation and coordination of medical, technical and socioeconomic data (national registration and record keeping of the population receiving home respiratory assistance)

4. Education of the patients and provision of general information
5. Development of national and international exchanges.

Each of the 33 regional associations functions administratively and economically independent from each other. However, they are organized with the same goals and objectives.

RESPONSIBILITIES AND ORGANIZATION OF THE REGIONAL HOME CARE ASSOCIATIONS

The organization of each regional association is basically the same, with all having a responsible physician, administrator and technician. In addition, most organizations have nurses on the staff.

Usually the association physician is part-time, and also works part-time in clinical practice. In most situations, he or she is responsible for the collection and review of patient medical data, training and education of technicians and nurses, the selection and trial of medical equipment and the initiation of new techniques. The physician is not responsible for home visits or medical decisions on patient care. The administrator is usually full-time and is responsible for managing the personnel and finances of the organization. This individual is the main contact between the regional organization, ANTADIR and the social security agency.

The role of the technician is to prepare, install and maintain all the medical equipment in the patient's home. These individuals provide 24 hour on-call support for equipment problems and repair. Nurses provide paramedical support in the home for the more technically dependent patients.

The responsibilities of the home care organizations are:

1. To establish a treatment plan for the patient, containing the physician's prescription and other necessary admin-

istrative information so as to obtain authorization from social security for payment.

2. To provide the patient with all necessary medical equipment and supplies, including the distribution of liquid oxygen.

3. To teach the patient and/or family how to use and maintain the equipment properly and to perform all necessary medical procedures, including changing the transtracheal catheters or tracheostomy tubes, where appropriate. If the patient or family is unable to assume responsibility for this level of care, local private nurses are taught how to perform these procedures.

4. To maintain the equipment in proper working order with systematic home visits for service and preventative maintenance every 2–6 months depending on the type of equipment and the level of patient dependency.

5. To provide 24 hour on-call service for equipment problems.

6. To provide paramedical supervision with systematic home nursing visits to ensure the patient and/or family continues to use the equipment properly. This includes checking patients, their compliance with treatment, SaO_2, proper fit of interfaces, adverse effects and equipment hygiene. In some cases services can include the monitoring of home nocturnal SaO_2 during respiratory assistance.

7. To maintain communication with referring physicians. Documentation of both technical and paramedical visits is sent to the referring physician and/or the patient's personal general practitioner. Any concerns arising from these visits are also directly communicated.

The regional association in Lyons – the ALLP (Association Lyonnaise de lutte contre la poliomyelite), one of the largest regional organizations, has 30 full-time employees and is responsible for 1500 patients treated at home.

PRESCRIPTION AND GUIDELINES

Prescription for HRC is the responsibility of a physician. All physicians can prescribe HRC, but the majority who initiate treatment are respiratory physicians, intensivists and paediatricians from both public and private practice. The prescription consists of a standard form containing administrative and medical data (diagnosis of the pulmonary disease, arterial blood gas tensions on room air, pulmonary function tests, haematocrit, symptoms of right cardiac heart failure, the details of the desired respiratory assistance).

LTOT is usually prescribed by respiratory physicians and is very decentralized. Guidelines for the prescription of LTOT are very precise and restrictive, in accordance with the recommeidations published after the NOTT and MRC studies for COPD patients [1,2,8].

HMV is much more centralized, using large hospital-based treatment teams. Intensive care units are also frequently involved – these may be private or public, but are mostly public. Guidelines for mechanical ventilation are imprecise, but are partly controlled by a list of acceptable aetiologies which inclued: restrictive patients, such as those with idiopathic scoliosis, sequelae of tuberculosis, neuromuscular disease and COPD. Patients should present with symptomatic chronic alveolar hypoventilation [9].

Guidelines for CPAP prescription have recently been initiated (April 1994) and require demonstration of the combination of an apnoea/hypopnoea index >30 per hour of sleep and excessive daytime sleepiness.

PAYMENT FOR HRC

HRC is paid for by the national health care system (social security). Obligatory contributions collected as payroll deductions from workers and employers finance social security. The National Health Care Financing Authority for Salaried Workers (CNAM), which works under the control of the Ministry of Health and Social Security, negotiates every year the rate of reimbursement that the local social security will pay for each day spent at home by a patient using HRC. Ten different rates are defined by the type of equipment and not by the type of disease. The calculation of the rate is complex, with an attempt made to establish the real cost of providing the therapy. The goal is also to maintain stability in the cost of HRC. To establish the rates, the social security includes the estimated real costs, the probable number of patients for the next year, the cost of operation of the organization, the inflation level, and the global financial result of the preceding year (avoiding a financial gain or deficit in view of non-profit status). The local social security section is responsible for administration, control (medical care by their own physician) and payment for HRC. The rate includes O_2 therapy and the electrical consumption of the equipment.

Costs vary between regions, despite the efforts of ANTADIR to standardize rates. The regional organizations are not equal, differing by their length of service, size, number of employees and balance of clientele (LTOT versus HMV).

In 1993, the national average daily rate varied betwen 44 FrF for LTOT by concentrator, 96 FrF for liquid O_2, 72 FrF for nasal positive pressure ventilation and 103 FrF for tracheostomy ventilation. The cost of LTOT and HMV is completely reimbursed by the social security, so that patients with chronic respiratory insufficiency have no individual financial responsibility. The rapid growth in CPAP prescriptions has recently created concern in the National Health Care Financing Authority. As a result, it has been decided to limit the prescription (guidelines), the suppliers (limited to the regional non-profit organization) and the reimbursement of CPAP. Social security will now reimburse only 65% of the daily cost of CPAP. The patient incurs the remainder of the cost personally or via individual private insurance.

The private system in France is usually managed by pharmacists and industrial companies who are required to provide the same service as the non-profit organizations. Their activity is mainly devoted to LTOT, especially liquid O_2 and more recently NIPPV. Private companies are rarely encouraged to take responsibility for severe cases such as tracheostomized ventilator-dependent patients. They are paid by social security, with a uniform national rate by therapy. Payment is usually 40% more than the regional association due to tax liability, debt obligation and the return of equity.

ORGANIZATION IN EUROPE

Much can be learned from reviewing the experience of HRC of different countries. Information is difficult to obtain, however, as only a few countries have national organizations and registers. Large discrepancies exist between countries, therefore 10 countries will be reviewed, eight of which were chosen primarily because of data availability though their participation in the European community. The other two countries, Sweden and Switzerland, provide interesting information on the length of experience of HRC. Sweden was markedly affected by polio epidemics. Switzerland utilizes the National Lung Organization for the distribution of HRC [6,10–14]. A summary of information regarding HRC in these 10 countries can be found in Table 16.1. The figures given in the table are estimates, not national statistics.

The first item in the table documents who can prescribe HRC. In countries where the prescription is limited to respiratory physicans, there seems to be a lower use of LTOT. The presence of national guidelines also contributes to a lower uptake, with the excepion of Spain, where guidelines were introduced very recently.

Reviewing the techniques used, it is surprising how many countries continue to use oxygen by cylinder which is more expensive

153

Table 16.1 Main information concerning organization of home respiratory care in ten European countries

	F	G	UK	I	B	NL	S	DK	SW	CH
Prescribers	Every physician	Every physician	P suggests and GP prescribes	P and I	P and I	Every physician	P and I	Varies from country to county	P, physician paediatrician	LTOT: GP and P HMV: P and I
National guidelines	For LTOT and CPAP	Yes	For LTOT	No	Yes	No	Yes	No	For LTOT	Yes
O_2 conc. (%)	85	90	60	20	62	15	9	81	90	70
Cylinder O_2 (%)	2	2	40	20	*	83	90	19	10	30
Liquid O_2 (%)	15	8	0	60	38	3	*	0	0	*
nPV (%)	1	4	22	15	1	15	1	1	1	0
NIPPV (%)	38	50	60	40	34	25	89	15	60	90
T-IPPV (%)	60	35	15	45	65	60	10	79	30	10
Supply and supervision of material	Regional assoc. CC	CC	LTOT: CC HMV: hospital	CC	CC or hospital	CC or centre for HMV	CC	CC	CC or hospital	National lung organization or CC
Patient home supervision	Nurse, technician	Physician	GP	Physician, nurse	Hospital	Nurse, physician, HMV centre	Nurse	Nurse, physician	National lung organization	National lung organization
Patients per 10^5 inhabitants										
LTOT	49	6	18	20	12	44	115	40	12	16
HMV	16	1	1	2	2	3	1	2	4	2
CPAP	13		3				19		10	

F, France; G, Germany; I, Italy; B, Belgium; NL, Netherlands; S, Spain; DK, Denmark; SW, Sweden; CH, Switzerland. Prescribers: P, respiratory physician; I, intensivist; GP, general practitioner.

CC, commercial company.

*Very limited use.

O_2 conc. 1, O_2 concentrator.

than oxygen concentrators. Equally surprising is the extensive use of liquid oxygen in Italy. This is most likely to be related to the high profile of commercial companies who, in an effort to promote their products, have been instrumental in developing programmes and education for HRC. A similar situation is occurring in France and, although this is may not be apparent from the table, if one looks at the percentage use of liquid oxygen in the private sector it is double that of the public (30% versus 15%). In contrast, in some countries liquid O_2 is unobtainable (England, Denmark and Sweden).

Because of the lack of national organization and the small number of patients affected, in comparison with LTOT, there is much less statistical information regarding HMV, the data being mainly estimates. Guidelines are almost non-existent. In Europe, there is relatively little experience of negative pressure ventilation (nPV). In addition, the interest has further decreased with the advancement of nasal intermittent positive pressure ventilation (NIPPV). NIPPV has increased access to home mechanical ventilation and this technique is widely used in Germany, UK, Sweden and Switzerland as well as in France, Italy, Holland and Belgium where the number of tracheostomized patients (T-IPPV) remains high. The relatively stable number of tracheostomized ventilator users in these latter four countries is probably related to the high survival rate of patients with restrictive disorders and to the fact that when NIPPV is unavailable, tracheostomy is used. This is rarely the case in other countries.

The supply of home respiratory equipment is provided by commercial companies in most countries. In some countries, however, there is cooperation between hospitals and regional associations for the purchase of more sophisticated equipment. Many countries report a need to improve the quality and consistency of home monitoring. Technical supervision is usually provided by the technicians of the commercial companies and/or the regional association. In general, technical monitoring is much more organized and consistent than home patient monitoring and supervision. Patient monitoring, when provided, is most frequently done by nurses and sometimes physicians from prescribing organizations or hospitals. With the technical sophistication of HRC and the necessary involvement of both technical and professional support, it is not surprising that the cost of HRC is high and without question cannot be provided without involving each country's national health system. In all countries represented, this is the main payment source for HRC. However, the level of cost and reimbursement of HRC differs widely between countries. Explanations for this can be found not only in variable medical practices but also in financial, social and political differences. One example can be found in the participation of the patient in the funding of CPAP. With the recent explosion in the detection of sleep apnoea and the general lack of adequate guidelines for the prescription of CPAP, some national health services are requiring patients to assume part of the financial responsibility for CPAP (France and Italy).

Lastly, the number of patients treated per 100 000 inhabitants varies markedly between countries, especially for LTOT. This cannot be explained by differences in the incidence of pulmonary disease but may be due to the differences in prescription habits and the information available to the physicians and the consumers. In addition, guidelines may be inadequately followed. Studies in Catalonia (Spain) and Denmark showed that in up to 50% of patients, the criteria for LTOT were not met. The level of prescription of LTOT in France also suggests excessive prescriptions [11].

In contrast, prescription of HMV seems abnormally low in all European countries by comparison with France. This can best be explained by the early development of HMV in France, particularly in chest wall disorders [3,4].

DISCUSSION

The main goals of home respiratory care have been outlined in Chapter 15. To some degree these goals have been met in selected groups of patients with CRI, e.g. mechanical ventilation especially for restrictive and neuromuscular patients, CPAP for sleep apnoea syndrome, LTOT for COPD.

Resources for health care are finite and much more work is needed to clarify the indications for HRC. To accomplish the appropriate selection of patients many consider it is necessary to have precise guidelines, regulated prescription national data collection, regular review of outcome data and international comparison of the results.

Competition between private and public HRC organizations has several diverse effects. The positive aspect is the potential for improvement in quality of care and control of prices. Adverse effects include the potential over-utilization of services and a tendency to use more complicated and expensive options than necessary. An example of this is the abuse of liquid oxygen prescriptions.

Finally, HRC needs to be organized and regulated. Information gathered nationally and/or internationally is more valuable than individual small experiences. Despite the problems of bureaucracy, including a decrease in flexibility, systemic national organization allows the extension of services to a greater number of patients as a lower cost, with the ability to standardize equipment, supplies and supervision. Organizations able to do complex as well as simple tasks generally have higher standards of care and are more flexible in the range of patients they can treat. The involvement of professional staff is essential to provide additional educational services which may improve patient compliance and raise the quality of care in general.

When used appropriately, there can be no doubt about the benefits of HRC. Our job as physicians is to work with out national health care systems to continue to define and develop the most efficient system of delivery of home care.

REFERENCES

1. Nocturnal Oxygen Therapy Trial Group (1980) Continuous or nocturnal oxygen therapy in hypoxemic chronic obstructive lung disease. *Ann. Intern. Med.*, **93**, 391–8.
2. Medical Research Council Working Party (1981) Long term domiciliary oxygen therapy in chronic hypoxic cor pulmonale complicating chronic bronchitis and emphysema. *Lancet*, **i**, 681–6.
3. Robert, D., Gerard, M., Leger, P. *et al.* (1983) La ventilation mecanique à domicile definitive par tracheotomie de l'insuffisant respiratoire cronique *Rev. Fr. Mal. Respir.*, **11**, 923–36.
4. Leger, P., Bedicam, J.M., Cornette, A. *et al.* (1994) Nasal IPPV. Long-term follow-up in patients with severe chronic respiratory insufficiency. *Chest*, **105**, 100–5.
5. Sullivan, C., Berthon-Jones, M., Issa, F. and Eves, L. (1981) Reversal of obstructive sleep apnoea by continuous positive airway pressure applied through the nares. *Lancet*, **1**, 862–5.
6. Fauroux, B., Howard, P. and Muir, J.F. (1994) Home treatment for chronic respiratory insufficiency: the situation in Europe in 1992. *Eur. Respir. J.*, **7**, 1721–6.
7. Muir, J.F., Voisin, C. and Ludot, A. (1992) Home mechanical ventilation (HMV) – National Insurance System (France). *Eur. Respir. J.*, **2**, 418–21.
8. Task Group SEP (1989) Recommedations for long term oxygen therapy (LTOT). *Eur. Respir. J.*, **2**, 160–4.
9. Donner, C.F., Howard, P. and Robert, D. (1993) Patient selection and techniques for home mechanical ventilation. *Monaldi. Arch. Chest. Dis.*, **48**, 40–7.
10. Rigaud Bully, C. (1994) Home mechanical ventilation: organisation in different countries, in *Home Mechanical Ventilation* (ed. Robert, D., Make, B.J., Leger, A.I. *et al.*) Arnette

Blackwell, Paris, 27–35.

11. Viskum, K. (1993) Organisation of professional care services with special reference to LTOT. *Monaldi. Arch. Chest. Dis.*, **48**, 453–7.

12. Howard, P. (1992) Home mechanical ventilation and respriatory care in the United Kingdom. *Eur. Respir. J.*, **2**, 416–17.

13. Donner, C.F., Pesce, L., Zaccaria, S. *et al.* (1993) Organisation of respiratory home care in Italy. *Monaldi Arch. Chest Dis.*, **48**, 468–72.

14. Goldberg, A.I. (1994) Technology assessment and support of life-sustaining devices in home care. The home care physician perspective. *Chest*, **105**, 1448–53.

Appendix A   Suppliers of ventilatory equipment

This list is not comprehensive, but contains many of the major suppliers.

NASAL VENTILATORS

BiPAP S, ST, STD models

Respironics Inc.
1001 Murry Ridge Drive,
Murrysville,
Pennsylvania,
USA

UK: Medic-Aid
Hook Lane,
Pagham,
Sussex PO21 3PP
Tel.: 01243 267321

BromptonPAC
AdaptorPAC

PneuPAC Ltd
Crescent Road,
Luton,
Beds LU2 OAH
Tel.: 01582 453303

Monnal D, DCC
DP90

Taema
6 Rue George Besse,
CE-80-92182 Anthony,
Cedex,
France

UK: Deva Medical Electronics
8 Jensen Court,
Astmoor Industrial Estate,
Runcorn,
Cheshire
Tel.: 01928 565836

Suppliers of ventilatory equipment

Nippy

Thomas Respiratory Systems
33 Half Moon Lane,
Herne Hill,
London SE24 9JX
Tel.: 0171 737 5881/5991

Lifecare PLV-100

Lifecare,
655 Aspen Ridge Drive,
Lafayette,
CO 80026-9341,
USA

Lifecare Europe GmbH
Postfach 20,
Haupstrasse 60,
D/8031;
Germany
Tel.: 8152 93060

UK: PneuPAC
address as above

Companion 2801

Puritan Bennett
4865 Sterling Drive,
Boulder,
CO 80301,
USA

UK: Puritan Bennett (UK) Ltd
Unit 1 Heathrow Causeway Estate,
152-176 Great West Road,
Hounslow,
Middlesex TW4 6JS
Tel.: 0181 577 1870

CPAP MACHINES

Sullivan CPAP Systems
Sullivan Autoset System

Rescare
82 Waterloo Road,
NSW 2113,
Australia

Rescare (UK) Ltd
68 Milton Park,
Abingdon,
Oxon OX14 4RX
Tel.: 01235 862997

160

Remstar

Respironics/Medic-Aid
Address as above

Revitalizer
Horizon Auto Adjust CPAP system
Surveyor compliance monitor

DeVilbiss Health Care
Airline,
Spitfire Way,
Heston,
Middx TW5 9NR
Tel.: 0181 765 1133

Tranquility series

Healthdyne Technologies
1255 Kennestone Circle,
Marietta,
Ga 30066,
USA

UK: Healthdyne Technologies
Stable Barn,
Collipriest,
Tiverton,
Devon EX16 4PT

MASKS, NASAL PLUGS AND HEADGEAR

Contour silicone masks
Full facemask, headgear, soft cap,
chinstraps

Respironics/Medic Aid
Address as above

Sullivan bubble masks
Headgear, chin strap

Rescare Ltd
Address as above

Healthdyne Soft Series mask
Nasal seals, headgear

Healthdyne technologies
Address as above

Nasal pillows (Adam Circuit)
Headgear

Puritan Bennett
Address as above

HUMIDIFIERS

Heat and moisture exchangers:
Portex ThermoVent 1200

Sims Medical Distibution
New Universal House,
303 Chase Road,
Southgate,
London N14 6JB

Suppliers of ventilatory equipment

Engstrom Flex (suitable for use with
with nasal pillow circuit)

S&W Vickers
Ruxley Corner,
Sidcup,
Kent DA14 5BL

Fisher & Paykel
Water bath HC100 heated humidifier

Rescare Ltd.
Address as above

NASAL BRIDGE PROTECTION

Granuflex hydrocolloid dressing

ConvaTec Ltd
Harrington House,
Milton Road,
Ickenham,
Uxbridge UB10 8PU

Spenco Dermal Pad

Spenco Medical (UK) Ltd
Burrell Road,
Haywards Heath,
West Sussex RH16 1TW.
Tel.: 01444 415171

PNEUMOBELT

Pneumobelt

Lifecare
Address as above

Thomas Respiratory Systems
Address as above

NEGATIVE PRESSURE SYSTEMS

Pumps:
NEV 100 negative pressure ventilator
Newmarket ENPV ventilator and
compact cuirass pump

Lifecare Europe
Address as above

Si Plan Electronics Research
Avenue Farm Industrial Estate,
Birmingham Road,
Stratford-upon-Avon,
Warwickshire

Cuirass shells
Pulmo wrap, Nu Mo suits, jackets
and ponchos

Lifecare Europe
Address as above

162

Hayek Oscillator and cuirass shells

Medicom Ltd
The White House,
Lodge Road,
London NW4 4DD
Tel.: 0181 203 9698

Tank ventilator (iron lung)

DHB Tools
Althorpe Street,
Leamington Spa,
Warwickshire CV31 2AU

PortaLung Inc.
401 East 80th Avenue,
Denver,
CO 80229,
USA

Rocking bed

RSP Medical
Care Direct,
St George's Road,
Semington,
Trowbridge,
Wiltshire BA14 6JQ

Appendix B   Useful contact addresses

Eurolung Assistance
F Smeets, MD
Centre Hospitalier de Saint-Ode,
6970 Tenneville,
Belgium.
Tel.: 32 84 455444

Network of European centres specializing in respiratory home care. Can provide list of members

International Ventilator Users Network
G.I.N.I., 5100 Oakland Avenue,
206 St Louis,
Missouri 63110-1406,
USA

Network of ventilator users and caregivers. Regular newsletter and advice forum

Breathe Easy
Contact: British Lung Foundation,
8 Peterborough Mews,
London SW6 3BL
Tel.: 0171 371 7704
for details of local branch

UK-based club for people with long-term breathing problems. Run by members

Scoliosis Association UK (SAUK)
2 Ivebury Court,
323-327 Latimer Road,
London W10 6RA
Tel.: 0181 964 5343

Regular newsletter, advice and publications for adults and children with scoliosis, and caregivers

The Muscular Dystrophy Group of
Great Britain and Northern Ireland
7-11 Prescott Place,
London SW4 6BS
Tel.: 0171 720 8055

Local branches, family care officers, advice, publications

Useful contact addresses

British Polio Fellowship,
Bell Close,
West End Road
Ruislip,
Middlesex HA4 6LP
Tel.: 01895 639453

Local branches. Advice and publications, especially regarding late effects of poliomyelitis

Motor Neurone Disease Association,
PO Box 246,
Northampton NN1 2PR
Tel.: 01604 250505

Local branches. Information, advice and practical help.

Index

Page number appearing in **bold** refer to figures and page numbers appearing in *italic* refer to tables.

167